SLAY THE GIANT

The Power of Prevention in Defeating Heart Disease

By
Elizabeth Klodas, MD, FACC

ISBN 13: 978-1-59397-076-8
ISBN 10: 1-59397-076-2
Library of Congress Catalog Number: 2008921596
Book design and typesetting: American College of Cardiology
Printed in the United States of America
Second Printing: 2009

12   11   10   09   5   4   3   2

This book provides practical information on the prevention of heart disease. It is not intended nor should it be used as a substitute for consultation with and advice from your physician. The opinions expressed in this book are solely those of the author and do not necessarily reflect the policy of the American College of Cardiology. No endorsement of any company or product is implied or intended.

Address all inquiries to:

Permission Department
CardioSmart
American College of Cardiology
2400 N Street, N.W.
Washington, D.C. 20037

For my husband Owen
and my children Alex and Kevin
— you fill my heart with joy.

Contents

*Visit **www.CardioSmart.org** for information on how to prevent heart disease and news on the latest treatment options*

About the Author

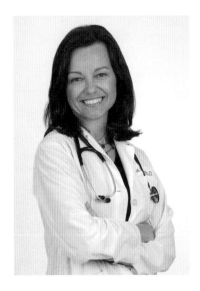

Elizabeth Klodas, MD, FACC, is a cardiologist working in Minneapolis, where she serves as Director of Cardiovascular Imaging at Center for Diagnostic Imaging.

Dr. Klodas received her doctorate from the University of Toronto in Ontario, Canada. She completed a comprehensive medicine internship at Toronto General Hospital and an Internal Medicine residency with the Mayo Graduate School of Medicine in Rochester, Minnesota. Dr. Klodas also spent five years studying cardiovascular diseases during fellowships with both the Mayo Graduate School, and Johns Hopkins School of Medicine in Baltimore, Maryland, focusing on noninvasive cardiology and echocardiography research.

Her professional interests include noninvasive cardiac imaging and valvular heart disease, but her true passion is heart disease prevention. Dr. Klodas directs the Cardiac Prevention Program at General Mills, and is beginning to work with several other employer and insurance groups to create robust prevention programs in the workplace.

Dr. Klodas' professional affiliations include the American College of Cardiology, American Heart Association, American Society of Echocardiography, and American Society of Nuclear Cardiology, of which she is a founding member of the Upper Midwest Working Group. She has authored numerous scientific articles and book chapters in her field, and serves on several professional committees, including CardioSmart, the patient education initiative at the American College of Cardiology.

Acknowledgments

This book arose as a consequence of crossing paths with one particular patient. But it would not have been possible without the assistance and support of numerous individuals. I would like to thank Rick Nishimura, Fred Bove, Richard Lewis, Suzy Hughes, and Steve Sjoblad for reviewing the manuscript, encouraging me, and providing constructive critiques. This book would not have been the same without your input. Rosemary Fruehling, for helping me navigate the publishing world and being the first to exclaim "Lizzie — you can write!" And Carl Pohlad, for constantly asking me if the book is finished yet. I would like to thank Mary Maier and Cathy Peterson — two outstanding nurses whose own passion for preventing heart disease helped propel my writing. And I would like to thank Jack Lewin, Steve Coy, Liz Wilson, Brad Ettinger, and Kristen Doermann at the American College of Cardiology for supporting my efforts and recognizing the need for a book such as this.

Milt Adams, you are a gem. And working with you at Beavers Pond Press has been a treat. Jennifer Manion and Terri Hudoba, your editing has made this work shine. And Morgan Bramlet, your artistic input brought the manuscript to life. I have truly been blessed to encounter so many wonderful people along this literary journey.

Most of all I would like to thank my parents, my husband, and my children. My mother and father have always believed in a balanced, healthful approach to life. They have always been advocates of prevention and have always challenged me to do the same. They also brought me up with a certainty that I could accomplish anything I put my mind to — and I hope I have lived up to their expectations. My husband and my children were left at times without a wife or mother as I clicked away on my laptop, literally possessed by writing this book. Your patience and encouragement are gifts I will treasure always. I love you with all my heart.

Foreword

Anyone hearing the current statistics on heart-related diseases and conditions in the United States is likely to feel a sense of concern, followed rather quickly by a sense of hopelessness. The rising rates of obesity and diabetes (both risks for coronary artery disease), especially among children, are certainly a cause for dismay. The members of the American College of Cardiology (ACC) feel that while a healthy concern is an appropriate, even necessary emotion, hopelessness is not. That's because there *is* hope and a chance for millions of people to live longer, healthier lives with a reasonable amount of effort and with the help of their medical team, including their cardiologist.

ACC — the primary professional medical society for 25,000 cardiovascular specialists in the United States and 10,000 from around the world — has been leading the way to optimal cardiovascular care and disease prevention since 1949. Fellows of the ACC (FACCs) are on the forefront of cutting edge research in cardiovascular disease and treatment. The ACC provides cardiologists and other health care professionals with the information and other resources they need to provide the highest-quality care to their patients. To this end, we promote health education and research, and we also develop and apply standards in cardiovascular care. As part of our mission, we are publishing this book by Dr. Elizabeth Klodas in an effort to educate the general public on the simple, yet effective, steps they can take to improve cardiovascular health and health overall.

In *Slay the Giant*, Dr. Klodas writes from her own heart with passion and a solid conviction that we *can* slay the heart disease giant by focusing on prevention. She breaks down a complex, often intimidating, subject into manageable bites, explaining medical terminology, providing pronunciation keys and simple definitions for those long and unfamiliar medical terms, and outlining key areas we all need to focus on to become — and remain — heart healthy. She also devotes a chapter each to what are perhaps the most talked about and least understood factors in heart health — HDL cholesterol, LDL cholesterol, and triglycerides. Dr. Klodas provides a simple way for readers to understand these factors and remember which one is which, and then demonstrates how to manage them for optimum health. Throughout this thought-provoking book, she interjects a welcome dose of humor, useful advice, and commonsense guidelines with which we can all live. Her book — which I know you will enjoy reading — is part of a larger effort on the part of ACC members to empower the public in their health care. We want to provide you with the tools and resources that will allow you to take charge of your health care in a dynamic way.

Recently, the ACC unveiled a new initiative called CardioSmart. A key piece of this is a Web site (http://www.CardioSmart.org) that serves the practical needs of patients, so they can better understand and manage their cardiovascular health. Dr. Klodas serves as the Web site's editor-in-chief. She and a medical advisory board provide content and also support physician-to-patient communication. The site is free of advertising content, which allows maximum focus on heart-related information and resources.

The CardioSmart Web site is designed to be patient friendly. Patients logging onto the site can —

- Access clear, easy-to-understand information and education resources;

- Participate in establishing a knowledge and experience base and developing a supportive online community;

- Gain a better understanding of critical guidelines and standards of care;

- More easily communicate with their cardiologist and better manage their health;

- Access moderated patient-to-physician and patient-to-patient forums; and

- Quickly locate ACC member cardiologists and health care providers.

Visitors to the CardioSmart site can learn how their heart works, the risk factors for heart disease, and ways to prevent the disease from occurring. They can also find up-to-date heart news (reviewed by board-certified cardiologists, accurately presented, without hype or factual distortions), and the CardioSmart Challenge, an online game designed to educate patients in an entertaining way. Two online forums — Ask a Cardiologist and Heart Patient Forum — provide an ongoing source of information and support for those managing their heart disease. A special area called Manage My Condition gives patients tools and guidelines to help them take a proactive role in their own care.

We invite you to visit the ACC Web site (www.acc.org) to learn more about the American College of Cardiology and the CardioSmart Web site to become and stay informed about your cardiovascular health. We also encourage you to use this book well, apply the advice, and share the information in it with those whom you love.

James T. Dove MD

James T. Dove, MD, MACC
Immediate Past President, American College of Cardiology

Introduction

The story behind the title

A long time ago, before I went to medical school, my father, who is also a physician, recounted a tale he had heard at a medical conference. The story summarized the status of medicine at the time. Even then, the tale struck me as having incredibly profound implications and, 20 years later, it continues to affect the way I view medicine and how I care for my patients. Here is that story.

A couple of doctors were passing by a river when they noticed an injured man floating by. He was gasping for air and crying out in pain. The doctors rushed into the river and pulled the man out. They tended to his wounds and eased his discomfort. Just as they were about to go on their way, two more injured people came floating down the river. And slightly upstream, five more bodies were visible. The doctors started pulling these individuals out, but knew they needed assistance. So they called for other doctors to come and help with the wounded.

The stream of injured grew larger and larger. And more and more doctors came to help. They built hospitals along the river's banks, and invented new methods to treat the patients more and more efficiently. Whole cities and industries sprung up in an effort to treat all the ill individuals. Thousands upon thousands of doctors flocked to the riverbank to help.

The doctors congratulated each other on every saved life. Their patients were grateful, and the doctors really felt like they were making a difference. Their inventions were much celebrated in the press, and their heroism was an inspiration to one and all.

But no matter how efficient and sophisticated the doctors became, no matter how many fancy machines or inventions they had, they could never quite keep up with the flow of patients. More and more kept floating down the river. The system was overwhelmed, the doctors were exhausted, and people were still dying.

Surprisingly, the doctors never walked upstream. If they had done this, they would have seen an angry giant clubbing people nearly to death and throwing them into the river. As it turns out, the real, lasting solution to the situation was not the complex one of investing time and resources into treating the injured, but rather a simple one: slay the giant.

Amazingly, this story, which highlights the pitfalls of treating disease instead of preventing it, is just as applicable to medicine today as it was in the previous millennium. We are so preoccupied with finding new ways to cure the sick that, as a society, we expend relatively little effort on keeping people healthy.

We have thousands of ways to treat patients who suffer form heart disease. We have fancy tests and miraculous procedures, specialized surgery and lasers and pacemakers. And yet we have accomplished relatively little in terms of reducing the number of people who develop heart disease — in fact, these numbers are *growing*. Heart disease is already the *number one* killer and disabler in the United States. And if you think it's an economic and social burden now, just wait until the baby boomers start hitting cardiologists' offices.

When it comes to heart disease, it's time for all of us to walk upstream.

This book is about slaying the giant.

The patient behind this book

Most patients affect physicians personally in some way, occasionally quite profoundly. I was happily working away in my practice, never even considering becoming an author, until the day I crossed paths with a young woman whom I'll call Ellen. Our encounter was so brief that I doubt she even remembers me, but Ellen left an indelible mark on my life. She was in her early 30s and had been diabetic since childhood. Her doctor had been treating her for asthma for almost a year, ever since she had been getting winded during physical activities. But her symptoms were not really improving.

She was out of shape and overweight. She did not know her own cholesterol levels and had "never paid attention" to her blood pressure numbers, though in fact she had elevated blood pressure readings and high cholesterol. Ellen's only health imperative had been to control her blood sugars. Because, as her doctors had told her, she was so young and (except for the diabetes) so healthy, she had never been placed on any medications other than those to control her blood sugar. Ellen didn't know that she was at very high risk for developing heart disease .

She was referred to me for a stress test. Lo and behold, her stress test findings were markedly abnormal! Actually, her test results were some of the most abnormal I had ever seen. Asthma was not the reason for her shortness of breath; she had an ailing heart. Ellen subsequently had an angiogram that revealed extensive blockages in all of her heart arteries, only some of which could be bypassed.

Her doctor was proud that he had finally diagnosed the problem. Ellen was grateful that her coronary disease was discovered "before it was too late." The surgeons saw her as a qualified technical success. I saw the whole situation only as a profound failure in heart disease prevention.

There was nearly nothing positive about Ellen's story. She had lived her life blissfully unaware of her risks. And her doctor had done nothing to reduce her chances of developing heart disease. By the time her coronary blockages were diagnosed, they were so advanced they couldn't even be fixed with surgery. And her chance of surviving into her 40s was almost nonexistent. Ellen was literally flailing in the river — she had actually been treading water for a very long time.

This is an extreme example, but I wish I could say it is unique. I also wish I could say it happened a long time ago and that things have changed — but this all took place last year. *Every single day* I cross paths with people who miss opportunities to prevent heart disease in themselves. And these individuals are literally putting their hearts on a one-way road to bypass surgery or early death. They take better care of their cars than they do of their own bodies. And they often blindly fail to question their care, or even seek preventative maintenance.

Ellen's experience really sparked my sense of urgency to write this book — something positive just had to come out of all of this. Her story was the straw that finally broke my back. I realized that, along the way, I had met far too many patients who lacked either the information or the motivation (or both) to affect their own outcomes. I knew it didn't have to be this way.

My goal in writing this book is to improve as many lives as possible, and prevent a lot of heart disease. My mission is to arm as many people as I can with the knowledge and motivation needed to improve their cardiovascular destinies.

But I will consider my mission accomplished if I can change just *one* heart's destiny. I hope it will be yours.

A few caveats

I wrote this book to help as many people as I could develop a good understanding of risk factors for heart disease — and how to reduce those risks.

The following pages contain synopses of discussions I have had with my patients, as well as the advice I have given them over the years. My goal is to give you that same map to get upstream.

I'm sure you will find within these pages some discussions that fit you to a tee and some pieces of advice you should definitely incorporate into your own life. But one size definitely doesn't fit all when it comes to medical advice — so be sure to evaluate your particular situation in consultation with your personal physician.

You will notice that I tend to use a lot of exclamation marks, italics, and bolded words and phrases in this book. When I speak about this topic I'm usually waving my arms around! I am *passionate* about promoting heart health and preventing heart disease, and I can't help conveying that passion on paper.

Because of the nature of the topic, you will be faced with some medical terms you might not know. Don't panic! I will try my best to make this topic approachable, understandable and applicable to your life. And the glossary at the end of the book should be helpful as well in defining unfamiliar terms.

This book is not meant to be a scholarly dissertation or a detailed biochemical explanation of heart disease. I want you to come away with important concepts, a framework and enough comprehension to make you an active and knowledgeable participant in your own care.

I am an adult cardiologist. That is, I specialize in the treatment and prevention of heart disease in adults. The contents of this book are directed toward preventing heart disease in adults. Your child's pediatrician is in the best position to advise you about optimal prevention strategies for your child.

The legal stuff: Any advice provided in this book needs to be interpreted within the context of your particular clinical situation. Your personal physician is the best person to help guide your care, including any prevention efforts. This book will help you be more informed and knowledgeable about heart disease and its risks so that you can have more meaningful and interactive discussions with your doctor, but it cannot and should not be construed as personal medical advice.

I hope that this book makes it possible for you to be your own best advocate. When it comes to heart health, you absolutely need to look out for number one!

E. Klodas M.D.

Elizabeth Klodas, MD, FACC
Editor-in-Chief, CardioSmart.org

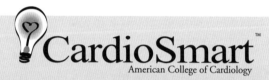

CardioSmart.org is the American College of Cardiology's online resource to enable individuals to work with their physicians to better understand, manage and impact their cardiovascular health. It includes the latest news on cardiovascular treatment options as well as information, tools and strategies to help prevent and control heart disease.

CHAPTER 1

Why You Should Care

Quit worrying about your health. It'll go away.
— ROBERT ORBEN

Y ou should care about your heart's health because even if you feel perfectly fine right this second, you could drop dead from a heart attack *today*. In fact, maybe right this minute.

OK — I am trying to scare you into action. But I'm also telling you the truth. Just because you don't show any symptoms of heart disease — or even have recently passed a stress test — heart disease is probably present within your body, and could "get you" out of the blue.

If you have risk factors that you are ignoring (or aren't even aware of), or you repeatedly make unhealthy lifestyle choices, you are literally *inviting* disaster.

Every day I see people live their lives in ways that virtually guarantee their developing heart disease. And truth be told, I've been guilty of the same behaviors from time to time. But those times are the exceptions rather than the rule for me, while the opposite is true for the vast majority of patients I see. This *must change.*

Next time you're at a restaurant, look around you. How many overweight people do you see? How many people eat obviously unhealthy food? How many clean their plates? How do you compare? Now, think of your neighbors and friends. How many people do you know who exercise every day? How many are as energetic as they were 10 years ago? How many look fit and lean? What about you?

Do you know what causes heart disease? What do you know about heart failure? Do you have any relatives who have suffered heart attacks or strokes or had bypass surgeries or angioplasties? Do you smoke? Do you have diabetes? Are you at risk for diabetes? What's your blood pressure? How much sodium do you consume? What's your cholesterol? (No, not your total cholesterol number: your LDL.) What's your HDL? Do you have metabolic syndrome? Have you ever had your lipoprotein A level evaluated? Do you know anything about C-reactive protein? Do you even know what I'm talking about??

Act now

Are you thinking: Whoa! Slow down!? And are you starting to feel that your lifestyle just might be out of control, and that you really don't have a great grasp of what causes heart disease and your level of personal risk? Well, the good news is (and this will make you feel better), you are not alone. The bad news is (and this makes me feel worse), *you are not alone.*

This book was written specifically to enhance your knowledge of heart disease — and to motivate you to make changes in how you live your life *today* — so that you don't have to worry about that giant throwing you into the river tomorrow.

The bottom line? All of our lifestyle choices and risk factors have cumulative effects. The sooner you start to make better choices, the sooner you get all your risk factors under control, the better long-term outcome you will have. You will not only live longer, but also live better. Aging does not have to be accompanied by disability. And it certainly doesn't have to be accompanied by cardiovascular disease.

Every choice you make, even if seemingly small, adds up. Every cheeseburger you consume affects your arteries and your waistline. Every cigarette you smoke is a cigarette ruining your heart. Every increase in blood pressure or cholesterol reading increases your chance of having a heart attack. Every walk you don't take reduces your endurance and resilience.

This book is about risk factors and choices, about heart disease and what you should understand about this modern-day health crisis. The more you know, the more you do, the greater your chances of survival. You should care — because this is about saving your life.

•

I hope that, by the end of reading this book, each one of you will say:

- *I will take back control of my life and make it better.*
- *I will stop putting junk in my mouth because I know that garbage in means garbage out.*
- *I will move my body every day.*
- *I will stop all harmful behaviors that are under my control.*
- *I will learn about heart disease and maintenance of heart health — because knowledge is power.*
- *I will acquire a good understanding of all my personal risk factors for heart disease and work hard to neutralize them as much as I can.*
- *I will do all of this because if I don't, I will die.*

Piece of Advice #1

Photocopy or transcribe the list above and put it in a place where you'll see it every day. You might need to put it in several places so that you *stay on task* with this. It really is a matter of life and death.

Learn more about preventing heart disease and how to make the right choices — visit www.CardioSmart.org

CHAPTER 2

Heart Disease 101

As I see it, every day you do one of two things:
build health or produce disease in yourself.
— ADELLE DAVIS

C ardiovascular disease is the number one killer and disabler of men and women. Did you hear me? The *number one* killer and disabler. And guess what — it is predominantly preventable.

Heart disease by the numbers

Nearly one million — deaths from heart disease in the U.S. every year — one death every *35 seconds*.

- 1 of 3 — people die of heart disease
- 120 to 150 years — our projected true lifespan, suggesting many of us will die at the halfway point.

Worldwide plague

Nearly one million people die of heart disease every year in the United States alone. That's equivalent to the population of a big city. Every year. That's one death every *35 seconds*.

At least one out of every three individuals will die of heart disease (actually more women than men die of heart disease each year), and all of us will have it to some extent, even if we die of something else.

Approximately 8,000 people reach the age of 60 every day in this country. Within the next 20 years, more than 100 million people will be over the age of 60 in the United States. If these individuals develop heart disease at current rates, the cost of their care could literally bankrupt this country. Have I got your attention yet?

And this is a plague not just affecting the United States. Cardiovascular disease is the number one killer and disabler in the entire Western world and, within a decade or two, it is expected to become the number one killer and disabler worldwide.

If you think that's impressive, what's really sobering is that heart disease doesn't just take the lives of elderly, frail individuals. It can take the life of an energetic 50-year-old man at the height of his career. Or a young mother with diabetes. It frequently strikes men in their early 60s and women in their early 70s. This might not sound too alarming (especially if you, the reader, are under age 40) unless you consider that many longevity specialists believe that our expected true lifespan probably approaches 120 — maybe even 150 — years. So people are dying at the halfway point of their lives. How could this be happening?

Silent killer

One reason is that heart disease is a stealth disease. It creeps up silently during a time in our lives when we feel positively immortal, and then makes a sudden appearance — usually in midlife — dramatically and often fatally. In fact, heart disease is different from many other diseases that affect us precisely because for the majority of its existence in our bodies, it is absolutely silent. But, as it turns out, even mild forms can be deadly. So waiting for heart pain before you start paying attention to this disease is *not* a workable strategy. You must jump on the prevention bandwagon right away — even if you have never thought about heart disease before. And by the way — it's *never* too late.

What is heart disease exactly? Well, many different disorders can affect how your heart functions. The majority of heart disease is related to coronary artery disease and to heart failure. We will examine each of these in turn, and concentrate on how to prevent these disorders in the remainder of this book.

A little warning: The following three chapters are rather "information intense" but not unapproachable. Take your time getting through this part of the book, and really make sure you absorb the concepts. You have to know what the giant looks like and what makes him tick. Understanding what you're up against is a vital part of preparing for battle!

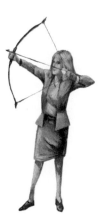

CHAPTER 3

CAD — It's Not Just Your Father's Disease

I don't want to achieve immortality through my work . . .
I want to achieve it through not dying.
— WOODY ALLEN

Coronary arteries are small blood vessels (slightly thicker than cooked spaghetti noodles) that provide the heart muscle with its own blood supply. (I will discuss the heart as a pump in the section about heart failure. Here I'm talking about the arteries that supply the heart muscle with vital nutrients and oxygen.)

Coronary arteries are just like arteries in the rest of your body. And your heart is predominantly a muscular organ. Just as the arteries in your legs supply blood to the leg muscles so you can walk or run, the coronary arteries supply blood to your heart muscle so it can beat.

Coronary artery disease (CAD)

CAD is the process by which "gunk" (sometimes referred to as "plaque") builds up in the walls of the coronary arteries. This gunk is made up of many different components including cholesterol, fat, inflammatory cells, calcium, muscle cells and fibrous tissue. If you have gunk in your arteries we (physicians) say that you have atherosclerosis. As more and more gunk builds up in the walls of the arteries, the lumen of those arteries (the hole or channel through which blood flows) becomes progressively smaller. Eventually, the lumen becomes so small that flow through one or more coronary arteries is insufficient to meet the demands of the heart muscle. This causes people to experience chest pain or shortness of breath when they're active, like when they're lifting heavy loads or exercising.

Demand outstrips supply

Here's what happens when you exercise: As you begin to get active (e.g., during a brisk walk), your leg muscles demand a more robust blood supply to get all the nutrients they need to allow you to move. This requires that your heart pump faster and with greater pressure to get more blood to the legs. In turn this means that your heart muscle works harder, and the heart muscle itself begins to make its own blood flow/nutrient demands.

If the demand outstrips the supply, your body can send you a signal. When running, you will eventually develop cramping in your calves as you continue to exert yourself. If your coronary arteries are too plugged up, you will eventually develop heart muscle cramping that you might feel as chest pain (angina) or unusual shortness of breath.

That's the general picture. The physiology behind all of this is a bit more complex.

As the heart muscle works harder, the coronary arteries respond by dilating, so that the artery lumen increases in size and more blood can flow through each artery to get oxygen and nutrients to the heart muscle. Using this mechanism, blood flow through normal heart arteries can increase up to fivefold. Even with strenuous exercise, we usually don't demand much more than a two- to threefold increase in flow over the baseline, so we have a big reserve built in.

When gunk progressively narrows the arteries, the arteries' ability to dilate enough to meet the demands of the heart muscle diminishes — the supply-demand balance tips and very strenuous activities become difficult. Since most people don't do much strenuous activity, the clogged arteries may go undetected.

As the gunk deposits get even worse, the supply-demand balance tips earlier, so that progressively less strenuous activities overwhelm the supply. Eventually, the interference with activities becomes noticeable enough that even rather sedentary people seek medical attention to get relief.

Think of highways and traffic patterns. If a city starts off with a four-lane highway and has the ability to open up 20 extra lanes on demand, it can handle a lot of traffic. In fact, most of the time the extra lanes won't be needed because the highway is pretty wide to begin with. So permanently closing one or two or even 15 of the lanes won't affect travel time too much, even at peak times. But if the highway narrows down to only a couple of lanes, and has none in reserve, traffic will snarl during rush hour. If the highway goes down to one lane, traffic will be horrible most of the time — and drivers will start to demand action from their city council.

Getting back to our arteries ...

Here's the most important point.

> *Because we have a big flow reserve built in, it takes a lot of gunk buildup to overwhelm the supply and demand balance — especially if we don't demand too much from the heart in the first place.*

Read the above paragraph again. This is a critical concept to appreciate.

It is not unexpected, therefore, that by the time patients feel chest pain or shortness of breath with activities, or by the time they have an abnormal stress test, they often have blockages that obstruct over 70 percent — sometimes over 90 percent — of the lumen of their arteries. That is, by the time patients have heart symptoms, or fail a stress test, they already have *advanced* coronary artery disease.

It was a shock!

Most people can recount the story of a relative, friend, or neighbor who was perfectly "healthy" until one day, all of a sudden, they needed quintuple bypass surgery. "It was a shock!" "But he was always so energetic!" "You'd never think it could happen to her!" If you understand the physiology of heart arteries and gunk buildup, these types of events should no longer surprise you. And you should start thinking about what might be accumulating in *your* arteries.

Luckily, the gunk doesn't build up overnight — it takes years, even decades, to develop severe blockages. So we have lots of opportunity to alter this process if we jump on the bandwagon early enough. But we cannot wait until we feel symptoms, because by then it might be too late to alter the course of this disease.

I've always found it amazing that it is relatively easy to get patients motivated to make changes once they've had angioplasty or bypass surgery, that is, once they've gotten to the cardiologist's office. But if you think about it — although preventive efforts are extremely important under those circumstances to avoid *future* need for similar procedures — in many ways these efforts are *way too late*. These individuals already have advanced coronary artery disease. They have floated way, way downstream and have been pulled out by all those doctors.

The challenge is to get people motivated to change their lives *before* they have been diagnosed with heart disease. People must be motivated to avoid the giant that wants to throw them in the river.

Lots of potholes

Another wrinkle in the story is that severe blockages are usually not responsible for heart attacks. In fact, study after study has shown that mild to moderate blockages are the usual culprits here. I'll talk about heart attacks and how they happen in the next chapter. For now, imagine the buildup of gunk as having two major effects on that highway of ours: (1) the progressive narrowing of the lanes, leading to the need for angioplasty and bypass surgery; and (2) the development of a lot of potholes in the road, making accidents (heart attacks) more likely.

So, when is the time to get serious about preventing heart disease? As early in your life as possible. In childhood. We know from autopsies performed on soldiers killed in the Korean and Vietnam Wars that even young individuals, young men in their early 20s, have evidence of plaque in their arteries. Some even have significant blockages. This process starts early and we influence its course every single day.

Piece of Advice #2

Live your life as if you already have heart disease. If you are an adult 40 to 50 years old, chances are very high that you already have some deposits of gunk in your arteries. You might not have severely narrowed lanes yet, but I bet you have some potholes. Be as vigilant about your health, your diet and your exercise regime as you can — as if your life depends on it. It does!

Piece of Advice #3

Impart healthful habits to your children. Even though children have amazingly resilient bodies, poor lifestyle choices are cumulative. If you live a healthier life and lead by example, you will not only be influencing your heart's destiny, you will also significantly affect the long-term health of the hearts of your little ones. For a superhighway to remain a superhighway, good maintenance is needed from the day the road is laid down.

For more information on how the heart works and what you can do to prevent heart disease, visit www.CardioSmart.org

CHAPTER 4

Facing the Facts

As for me, except for an occasional heart attack,
I feel as young as I ever did.
— ROBERT BENCHLEY (1889–1945)

Two-faced CAD

T here is something very important about CAD that you have to understand. As it turns out, this disorder has two faces. One is the progressive, generally slow accumulation of gunk in our arteries that eventually causes severe blockages leading to symptoms. This is the process we have been talking about so far, and risk factors for this occurring include:

- Smoking
- High blood pressure
- Cholesterol abnormalities
- Diabetes
- Inactivity

- Poor diet
- Excess weight
- A family history of heart disease
- Increasing age

Doctors have understood this process well for a long time, and many treatment options, from medications to angioplasty to stents to bypass surgery, exist to treat it. These are not necessarily options you would want to volunteer for, but they are options — and pretty good ones — if you need them. As you now know, this face of coronary disease is based on a large amount of gunk accumulating within the walls of the arteries.

Many patients assume that this process carried to the extreme (complete occlusion of the artery) is what causes heart attacks. Actually, this is not the way heart attacks happen. As I mentioned in the previous chapter, mild and moderate blockages cause the vast majority of heart attacks. So heart attacks happen by a different mechanism — this is the other face of coronary artery disease.

Endothelium attack

The other face of coronary artery disease is that of endothelial dysfunction and plaque instability. Endo-what? Plaque-huh? The **endothelium** (en-dough-THEEL-yum) is the innermost lining inside a coronary artery. This very thin, delicate layer of cells covers up the tissues making up the artery wall — much like skin covers the tissues of our hands, for example. The endothelium is the vital barrier between the blood flowing through the coronary artery lumen and the contents of the artery wall.

As gunk builds up inside the artery walls — and here's the major point — *any* amount of gunk — the endothelium becomes more vulnerable to injury or breakdown or sloughing. Think of the endothelium as getting stretched or deformed by the expanding gunk underneath, so that this protective barrier is thinned and more prone to disruption. Imagine the walls of a balloon expanding beyond capacity. You know what happens.

I'm going to repeat this for emphasis:

> *The presence of any coronary artery disease makes the endothelium vulnerable to injury.*

So, plaque might not build up silently after all. Sometimes plaque deposits (even minor ones) will burst open into the lumen of the artery — like a boil bursting — because the protective layer gets stretched beyond its limit.

Uncontrolled risk factors make the plaque deposits even more unstable and hence much more likely to burst open. You can think of uncontrolled risk factors behaving like little pins, poking the weakened endothelium, markedly increasing the chance that this stretched covering will burst.

So, for emphasis:

> *Uncontrolled risk factors are toxic to the vulnerable endothelium and increase the chance for plaque rupture.*

This has huge implications.

The clot that blocks

If the endothelium breaks down, the raw tissue underneath is exposed to the inside of the coronary artery. It's like if you sloughed a bunch of skin off your hand, or burst a boil, and the raw tissue underneath became exposed to the air. The body's automatic reaction would be to try to heal that area of exposed, raw tissue. So a scab would form on your hand to protect the injured area from the environment. The scab acts as a temporary barrier, giving the injured tissues a chance to heal and the skin time to grow back.

The story is similar with coronary arteries. When you slough off or break down an area of your endothelium "skin" or burst a plaque "boil," the body recognizes this as an injury and tries to fix it. The body responds by making a little blood clot at the site of injury to cover the raw area so that it has a chance to heal over and the endothelium has a chance to grow back. That blood clot is the artery's equivalent of the scab on your hand.

But remember that coronary arteries are small blood vessels, only slightly larger than spaghetti noodles. So if the blood clot is big enough, it can completely block flow through the coronary artery — an inadvertent, bad consequence of an initially self-healing process. A clot in a coronary artery can severely restrict or even cut off the flow of nutrients to the heart muscle. This is how a heart attack happens: by a sudden change in blood flow within a coronary artery.

A clot's progress

- A heart attack happens because a clot forms inside a coronary artery, disrupting blood flow to the heart muscle.

- The blood clot forms in reaction to the endothelium breaking down or plaque bursting.

- The endothelium is more prone to breaking down when *any* gunk is present in the wall of the coronary artery.

- Plaque is much more likely to become unstable or burst in the setting of uncontrolled risk factors.

This is why you have heard of cases in which someone passes a stress test with flying colors on Monday and then drops over dead on Wednesday. That person did not have significant blockages (so they passed the stress test), but they had vulnerable endothelium or unstable plaque that broke down and caused the heart attack. I mentioned earlier that it takes quite a bit of buildup (blocking over 70 percent of the lumen) to start to overwhelm the supply-demand balance. Therefore, it takes a lot of buildup to result in an abnormal stress test (which assesses that balance).

So it's not just the severe blockages we should be worrying about: *any* amount of gunk is a problem.

Can you see now how a lifelong runner or athlete at the peak of his career might die suddenly of a heart attack? Bottom line: unstable plaque can take anyone down.

People who have extensive coronary disease (and fail a stress test) have a greater risk of having a heart attack because, in general, they have more gunk in their arteries, more of their endothelium is at risk for breaking down and more of their plaque could be unstable. They also often start off with smaller coronary lumens, so even a small clot can plug up the flow.

Still with me? There are several corollaries to all of this.

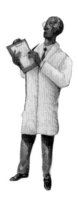

Reining in risk

- A normal stress test, though reassuring and a good baseline, does *not* mean that you don't have *any* coronary artery disease.

- A normal stress test result is *not* a free pass to making poor lifestyle choices or to ignoring any risk factors you may have for developing heart disease.

- Even if you do not have any symptoms of heart disease, the process may be progressing inside your body and you could be faced with a sudden, major, life-altering event if you continue to ignore any **risk factors** you may have.

- The same risk factors that cause gunk to build up inside our arteries also make the endothelium more vulnerable to breaking down and make plaque unstable. Here's that list again:

    — Smoking
    — High blood pressure
    — Cholesterol abnormalities
    — Diabetes
    — Inactivity
    — Poor diet
    — Excess weight
    — A family history of heart disease
    — Increasing age

- Controlling your risk factors not only prevents the need for bypass surgery and stents, but also prevents the occurrence of heart attacks.

When we control risk factors, we reduce the number of pins circulating in our blood streams. The fewer the number of pins, the lower the chance that one of the pins will poke a stretched area of lining and the lower the risk of a heart attack. The fewer risk factors, the lower the chance of accumulating more gunk in the walls of the arteries and creating traffic jams, and the lower the chance of requiring heart-artery stents or bypass surgery in the future. *So, no matter where you start from, control your risk factors to ensure your survival and assure good quality of life.*

I hope you feel the sense of urgency that I am trying to convey.

An aspirin a day

You may have noticed that when patients have documented coronary artery or vascular disease or have diabetes, doctors routinely place them on aspirin therapy (usually 81 mg/day — the equivalent of a "baby" aspirin). This is because aspirin is a mild blood thinner, helping to prevent blood clots from forming if plaque breaks down or ruptures — or at least helping ensure that the clot that forms is small enough that it doesn't completely cut off blood flow. Aspirin has no effect on cholesterol levels, blood pressure or the amount of plaque buildup. It's importance lies in its ability to thin the blood.

It's not unusual for doctors to recommend that men over the age of 50 and women over the age of 60 take a daily aspirin — even if they don't have a previous history of heart problems or stroke — because chances are very high that their arteries have some plaque, the substrate that might cause trouble.

If you are currently not taking aspirin but fit into one or more of the categories of patients who might benefit from this therapy, please don't run out to one of those warehouse stores and buy that giant bottle of aspirin just yet. Talk to your doctor first to make sure it is OK for you to be taking aspirin regularly. Even though the preventative amount is a "baby" dose, aspirin is a drug with potential for complications. You want to be reasonably certain that this prevention step is right for you.

Stroke happens

By the way, a stroke happens in a way very similar to the way a heart attack happens. A stroke doesn't happen because an artery in the neck occludes slowly and completely over time. It happens because the endothelium in a neck artery breaks down or a bit of plaque bursts and a blood clot forms at the site.

The main difference between a heart attack and a stroke is that the neck arteries have significant redundancy built in (there are four separate arteries that supply blood to the brain, and they interconnect in a web of medium-sized blood vessels in the skull). Neck arteries are also large arteries compared to those of the heart, so it is unusual for a blood clot to be big enough to completely obstruct a neck artery. Rather, in the case of stroke, it is probably more common for the blood clot that has formed in one of the neck arteries to break off and travel downstream, occluding a much smaller artery in the brain, or for a clot to form in a vulnerable, small artery within the brain, beyond the redundant web of interconnected blood vessels.

The endothelium in the neck and brain arteries (and in all arteries for that matter) is the same endothelium that is found in the coronary arteries. The plaque that builds up in the coronary arteries is the same plaque that builds up in other arteries in our bodies. Any risk factors that could cause the endothelium or plaque to be more vulnerable in the heart arteries will make endothelium and plaque more vulnerable *in general.*

Atherosclerosis (the general term for the accumulation of gunk or plaque) is a *systemic* disease. That is, if blockage or buildup is found somewhere in *one* artery, chances are very high that blockages or buildup exist *elsewhere.* So when you protect yourself from heart disease, you also protect yourself from stroke and from peripheral vascular disease (blockages in the arteries of the legs, aorta, penis and so forth — gentlemen, you should be getting very motivated! In all seriousness, peripheral vascular disease is one of the most common causes of impotence).

Time is muscle

Earlier I mentioned that there are many treatment options for the first face of CAD (the slow, progressive buildup of gunk). For the second face — heart attack — our options are much more limited, not necessarily by lack of technology or medications — but by lack of *time*.

When a heart attack happens, heart muscle begins to die almost immediately, and the chance of saving heart muscle falls off precipitously the longer the blood supply to the heart remains cut off. The chance of staving off major heart muscle injury is best if the blood supply to the heart muscle is restored within minutes to an hour of the start of symptoms.

Heart muscle doesn't grow back very well — this is why you want to save as much of it as quickly as possible. And when you damage a large part of your heart, the pumping function deteriorates. As a consequence, the heart becomes less able to meet the demands of your body's other tissues, limiting both what you can do and your lifespan.

After four hours from the start of a heart attack, there is still a chance of saving some, but not necessarily a majority, of the heart muscle. After 12 hours, the chances of saving heart muscle are so remote that heroic measures (like giving powerful clot-buster medications or performing emergency angioplasty) are generally not expected to make much of a difference and are not routinely used.

In short, *time is muscle.*

The best way ...

- to save heart muscle is never to have a heart attack — never to need all those doctors assembled at the river's edge.

- to enssure that you never have a heart attack is to begin an all-out prevention campaign for yourself. Today.

But if you really need a more sobering thought, you should know that a heart attack doesn't always give you time to respond. *A heart attack can kill you within a couple of minutes.* Heart muscle that is suddenly cut off from its oxygen and nutrient supply can scramble the natural electrical impulses that travel through it — resulting in rapid and deadly heart rhythms.

Half of all heart attacks result in instant death. This is not how you want to find out you have a problem.

CHAPTER 5

Failure to Perform

Men are born to succeed, not fail.
— Henry David Thoreau (1817–1862)

Heart failure is the general term given to a group of disorders in which there's an imbalance between the effectiveness of the heart's ability to pump blood and the body's demands. Another imbalance! This time we are not talking about disorders of the heart's arteries but of the heart muscle itself.

We're switching gears here. For now, don't think about those cooked-spaghetti-noodle blood vessels. Think about the heart purely as a muscular pump that moves blood around the body. As you exercise, that muscle has to pump faster and harder.

Heart pump

The heart pump has two important phases that make up the **cardiac cycle**, the entire series of events that takes place from heartbeat to heartbeat.

The first phase is **systole** (CIS-tuh-lee), the actual ejection of blood from the pumping chambers of the heart. This phase depends upon heart muscle contraction and results in the squeezing of blood out of the heart to the body. If your heart's ability to contract is impaired, your heart will not be able to pump enough blood forward to meet your body's demands, and you will not be able to do the things you want to do. Over time, especially if the dysfunction remains untreated or progresses, you will become breathless when doing activities. Your ankles will swell. Fluid will build up in your lungs. And you will die ahead of your time.

The second phase of the cardiac cycle is **diastole** (die-AHS-tuh-lee), the period during which the heart muscle relaxes and the heart cavity fills with blood. If the heart muscle becomes stiff, it cannot relax well. If it cannot relax well, it cannot properly fill with blood, making less blood available within the heart cavity to be pumped forward. So even if contraction/systole is fine, poor relaxation will lead to your heart not being able to pump enough blood forward to meet your body's demands — and you will not be able to do the things you want to do. Just as with systole, over time, especially if the dysfunction remains untreated or progresses, you will become breathless when doing activities. Your ankles will swell. Fluid will build up in your lungs. And you will die ahead of your time.

Problems with either systole or diastole (or both) will result in the same constellation of symptoms. And the same bad outcome — a shorter life span.

In case you are panicking right now because your ankles tend to swell or you get winded walking up a couple flights of steps, know that there are many reasons why people develop these symptoms. And often these reasons are not life threatening or associated with bad outcomes. Not all ankle swelling is due to heart failure, and not all shortness of breath is related to heart disease. But if you have these symptoms and have never discussed them with your doctor, make an appointment to get evaluated. If your car were making a funny noise, you'd probably take it in to the shop. Most little clunks require just minor adjustments and don't represent big problems. But occasionally, they point to big issues with the engine.

Many people who develop heart failure have coronary artery disease and have sustained heart muscle damage due to one or more heart attacks. Heart damage due to a heart attack will affect systole/contraction. So when you prevent coronary disease, you prevent heart attacks and heart failure.

Muscle bound

But you can develop heart failure without having severe or advanced CAD. **Hypertension** (high or uncontrolled blood pressure) on its own will lead to heart failure over time. Hypertension causes heart failure by consistently putting a strain on the heart muscle.

The heart, when it deals with blood pressure, is like a weight lifter lifting weights. As the weight lifter trains with heavier and heavier weights, the weight lifter's body adapts by building up the arm, leg, and back muscles. Similarly, as the average blood pressure rises, the heart muscle adapts by becoming thicker. So far, so good.

Over time, the weight lifter loses flexibility as he continues to build muscle bulk. In the heart, over time, increased stiffness begins to accompany heart muscle thickening, and the heart becomes "muscle bound." This is an unwanted development, and affects diastole. As heart relaxation becomes more and more compromised, heart failure develops.

But even if relaxation is not affected to a major degree, contraction can also become affected over time. If the weight lifter continually lifts heavy weights without any breaks, he eventually gets tired; he has to put the weights down and take a rest to allow his bulky muscles to recuperate. Same with high blood pressure: As the pressure remains elevated (for years), the heart muscle, even if thickened, eventually gets tired of lifting that weight and so begins to fail. The heart-pumping function (contraction/systole) can deteriorate, and this too translates into reduced overall stamina and shortness of breath and ankle swelling.

Hypertension accompanies excess weight and inactivity, as well as a high-sodium diet. Generally, you can't feel your blood pressure — so unless you check and monitor it, you might not know that you're walking around with a pressure that is too high. Walk around with high blood pressures for too long, and your heart will start to fail. And you will die ahead of your time.

Double-edged sword

Obesity and diabetes (both risks for coronary artery disease) have also been shown to adversely affect diastole. Preventing these disorders will also lower the chances that you develop heart failure.

Excessive alcohol consumption can lead to heart failure. I'm not talking about when you have "one too many" at an occasional party. I'm talking about the regular consumption of large amounts of alcohol. Alcoholics are very much at risk for this complication. Alcohol can be toxic to heart muscle, which is one of the reasons physicians are often skittish about recommending alcohol consumption to their patients. On the other hand, alcohol consumption in moderation has been repeatedly shown to reduce cardiovascular risk. Just remember, *moderate consumption means one to two alcohol-containing drinks per day:* one for women or smaller adults, two for men. (One drink is defined as 12 ounces of beer, 5 ounces of wine, or 1 1/2 ounces of spirits or hard liquor, such as gin or whiskey.) If you regularly consume more than this, you may be putting your heart muscle at risk. Alcohol truly is a double-edged sword.

Many other disorders can affect heart muscle function, but these are much less common than hypertension and coronary artery disease. If you prevent CAD and treat or prevent hypertension, you prevent the vast majority of life-limiting heart disease.

How we go about preventing these diseases is the focus of the remainder of this book.

Pep talk

If you're starting to get a little depressed about all of this — please don't despair! Untill now, this book has hopefully helped you understand what you are up against. Begin making changes *today* so you don't become another statistic —

- You may well have already developed some coronary disease.
- The process is to some extent reversible, and the road to heart failure can be avoided with appropriate lifestyle changes.
- These may not be small changes.
- But I promise you — they are attainable.

Regardless of your health at the moment, you *can* improve your well-being and increase your life span! To start right now, simply turn the page!

To learn more about how the heart works and what you can do to prevent heart disease, visit www.CardioSmart.org

CHAPTER 6

Cholesterol Basics

Is it better to be the lover or the loved one?
Neither, if your cholesterol is over six hundred.
— WOODY ALLEN

Our bodies need **cholesterol:** It is a necessary building block. For example, it is an integral component of the cell membrane, the wall of every cell within the body. So for simplicity's sake, you can think of cholesterol as tiny bricks that the body uses to build all its walls. Blood transports cholesterol around the body as particles, and those cholesterol particles are made primarily in the liver. Cholesterol eventually becomes incorporated into the tiny cell walls as required. But excess cholesterol that is not needed by the body's cells can get deposited into the walls of arteries, leading to the development of blockages.

Excess cholesterol is one of the most clearly linked and significant risk factors for heart disease.

Knowing your cholesterol level is therefore one of the most basic and essential cornerstones of understanding your personal risk of future heart problems.

Heart of the matter

Your cholesterol levels usually deteriorate when you —

- Age.

- Eat poorly.

- Sit on the couch.

- Inherit unlucky genes.

- Lose estrogen (in women).

- Get fat.

Cholesterol profile

A blood test can measure your cholesterol levels and general guidelines spell out what those cholesterol levels should be. Many factors influence your total cholesterol level, as well as the various components that make up your cholesterol "profile" (the more detailed analysis of the various cholesterol particles that make up the total cholesterol number). Here are some of those factors:

- **Age.** Cholesterol levels tend to be lower in younger individuals, since they are quickly using up the bricks to build more and more cell walls in their growing bodies. (Interestingly, patients with advanced cancer tend to have extremely low cholesterol levels because the rapidly multiplying cancer cells are quickly using up the supply of circulating bricks.) As we age, cholesterol levels tend to go up as the need for bricks and new walls goes down. So ... get older and your cholesterol levels go up.

- **Diet** can have a big impact on cholesterol levels. Many people assume that their blood cholesterol levels will go down if they just cut their cholesterol consumption. This is not necessarily the case. *The vast majority (over 80 percent) of cholesterol in your blood stream is manufactured internally by your liver and is not related to cholesterol in the food you eat.* So, the effect of diet is much more complex and has more to do with the overall picture rather than with one particular dietary component. It's not just about cutting down fat either (more on that later). So ... eat poorly and your cholesterol levels go up.

- **Exercise** can affect cholesterol levels positively. Moving your body and staying fit dramatically impacts your cholesterol profile. To build new cells (growing muscles) and repair old ones and to combat the physical stress of exercise, we use up more building materials. So ... sit on the couch and your cholesterol levels go up.

- **Genetics** plays a tremendous role regarding cholesterol. Each of us is born with a blueprint that tells the body exactly how and when to make cholesterol. Most of the time, that scripted manufacturing process can be affected (sometimes quite dramatically) by lifestyle changes. But sometimes, no matter what an individual does, his or her cholesterol profile remains completely, absolutely, and frustratingly immovable. So ... inherit unlucky genes and your cholesterol levels stay up.

- **Estrogen.** Speaking of genetics, women tend to have a bit of an advantage over men, at least for a while. Prior to menopause, higher estrogen levels can favorably influence the cholesterol profile, if not so much the total cholesterol number. Estrogen tends to raise HDL levels — levels of the good cholesterol — and this is thought to be protective. Once women go through menopause, however, anything masked by the estrogen effect becomes exposed. Women who undergo removal of both ovaries (as part of a total hysterectomy, for example) prior to natural menopause will experience the same cholesterol alterations. So ... lose estrogen and your cholesterol profile gets worse.

- **Weight** can influence the numbers. Given the above discussion, one would think that as people get bigger, they need to make more or bigger cell walls and their cholesterol levels would drop. In theory this is correct, but in practice, as we gain weight we progressively and negatively change the biochemical makeup of our bodies, and those changes far surpass any "positives" we might realize from a more or bigger cell wall standpoint.

One of the major changes that occurs with weight gain is that our bodies generate progressively higher levels of insulin. **Insulin** is a storage hormone that allows us to store all the food (especially carbohydrates) coming in, in anticipation of the "lean times" ahead. (In the Western world, those lean times never come, at least not for most of us!) Insulin levels initially go up in overweight people because when more food is consumed, more insulin is released in response. Over time, cells in the body become less and less sensitive to the insulin that's always around, so that the body needs to manufacture more and more of it for the same net effect. Even if overweight people eat less, the relative rise in insulin levels will be higher for *any* food amount ingested. Because insulin is a storage hormone, it shifts our general biochemistry to storage mode, causing levels of bad cholesterol (LDL, the storage form) to go up, while levels of good cholesterol (HDL, the elimination form) go down. And triglycerides (sugar/fat storage particles) go up, often way up. Thus, even if the total cholesterol doesn't change much, the components making up that total can be dramatically altered for the worse. So ... get fat and get a bad cholesterol profile.

Numerology

So how do you know if your cholesterol numbers are up to snuff?

When you get your cholesterol checked, you are given at least a total cholesterol number. Most of the time, the cholesterol check not only gives you your total cholesterol number, but also the numbers for your HDL (good cholesterol), LDL (bad cholesterol), and triglyceride (TG, a mostly fatty particle with some cholesterol in it) levels. The amounts of HDL, LDL and

TGs make up the total cholesterol number and are related to each other in the following formula:

$$\text{Total cholesterol} = \text{HDL cholesterol} + \text{LDL cholesterol} + (\text{TG}/5)$$

Usually, the total cholesterol, HDL cholesterol and triglycerides are literally measured, while the LDL is calculated. The formula falls apart once TG levels are very high (over 400). Under those circumstances, the LDL cholesterol must be measured directly, requiring more specialized laboratory capabilities.

When you ask people who have had their cholesterol checked, most can tell you their total cholesterol number. But the total cholesterol can be made up of a lot of different combinations. For example, it may be composed of a lot of good cholesterol, a little bad cholesterol and moderate TGs; or a little good cholesterol, a lot of bad cholesterol and high TGs. The total number can be *exactly the same* in both circumstances. So the total cholesterol number gives you very little information about your actual risk profile. It is, for all intents and purposes, a fairly useless piece of information.

When it comes to knowing your cholesterol numbers, forget the total! This number does not help you. If during a cholesterol screening at work or at a health fair you were given your total cholesterol number, understand that you are not much farther ahead in terms of defining your cardiovascular risk. If this — your total number — is all you know about your cholesterol, talk to your doctor about getting a more detailed evaluation.

OK, so what should you know? *You should know (and understand) all three of the numbers that make up the total.* No shortcuts, no excuses. You know your telephone number, your social security number — your cholesterol numbers are in the same league. They are that important.

Now we need to discuss the different types of cholesterol particles. Don't worry: It's not as complicated as you might think.

CHAPTER 7

The Good — HDL

It's a good thing.
— Martha Stewart

HDL (high-density lipoprotein) is often referred to as the good cholesterol. You can remember that HDL is the **H**appy cholesterol and that you want your HDL number to be **H**igh. You can think of HDL cholesterol as garbage trucks. These particles are not depositing cholesterol in your arteries, but rather are removing it from your system. The higher the HDL cholesterol the better. You want as much of your cholesterol as possible to be on its way out of your body rather than finding a place to park in it.

When over 40 is good

Everyone's HDL cholesterol level should be above 40 mg/dL (you don't have to remember the units, just the numbers). Premenopausal women should have an HDL cholesterol well over 50 mg/dL. At the present time, one out of every four Americans has an HDL number below 40 mg/dL.

An HDL value exceeding 67 mg/dL in women and 53 mg/dL in men is considered a "negative risk factor," meaning it's like having a bit of an insurance policy against heart disease. Low HDL numbers, especially values below 37 mg/dL for men and 47 mg/dL for premenopausal women are a potent risk factor for developing early or aggressive heart disease.

HDL cholesterol levels can be very difficult to budge, but changes can be made.

I've already discussed the role of estrogen and menopausal status in women (HDL levels tend to be higher in women who are producing estrogen). It's therefore not surprising that one of the biggest hopes for preventing heart disease in women had been hormonal supplementation following menopause. For many years this was believed to be the "magic bullet" for women, and when women received estrogen supplements, we indeed saw their HDL numbers go up.

Unfortunately, modern medicine is not that good at replicating nature, and any benefits seen in cholesterol profiles were outweighed by higher rates of heart attacks and overall mortality in hormonally supplemented women (probably due to a greater propensity for blood clot formation). Studies have proven controversial; nevertheless, in several large trials hormone supplementation did not reduce the risk of heart disease. This was a big surprise for doctors, but the data so far appear consistent and reproducible, and at this time hormone supplementation cannot be viewed as a fail-safe method for preventing heart disease — and certainly not as a reasonable method to raise HDL levels.

HDL Basics

Optimal HDL level:

Over 53 mg/dL for men; over 67 mg/dL for premenopausal women
(this is often averaged to 60 mg/dL for everyone; bottom line —
the higher the better!)

Acceptable HDL level:

Over 40 mg/dL for men and postmenopausal women; over 50 mg/dL
for premenopausal women

Get help!

Under 37 mg/dL for men and postmenopausal women, under 47 mg/dL
for premenopausal women (this is often averaged to 40 mg/dL for
everyone; bottom line — the higher the better!)

Exercise raises HDL levels

One of the best ways to raise your HDL is to exercise regularly. Both
aerobic (cardio) and strengthening (weight-training) exercise improves HDL
levels. Doing some exercise every day is the goal. The least you should do
is a half hour of aerobic activity at least four days a week, and a half hour
of strengthening exercise at least two days a week. According to the latest
recommendations, moving your body for at least 60 to 90 minutes daily is
ideal. If this is not workable for you, at least *try* for that half-hour minimum.

You **must** move your body every day. Exercising should be as much
a part of your day as eating a meal or brushing your teeth. If you're not
exercising now, you can make exercise a habit. We all have different excuses
why we don't exercise — but each day that goes by without your taking care
of yourself is a day wasted, as far as your heart is concerned. Remember, it's
all cumulative!

A word here to you avid exercisers, especially if you run marathons or are otherwise in an elite athlete category. Should you stop exercising or diminish the intensity of your workouts significantly (even if this occurs gradually over time), be aware that your cholesterol profile may change dramatically. So, if during your peak years you had a stellar profile but you have slowed down (even though you may still be doing far more than most of us mortals) and haven't gotten a cholesterol check lately, go get one just to make sure you're as biochemically stellar as you used to be.

Another word of caution. I have seen many patients who, because they have been very physically active, have ignored their abnormal cholesterol readings, assuming that being fit makes up for bad cholesterol numbers. It does not. *Physical activity and cholesterol levels are separate risk factors.* Being physically active *can* improve your cholesterol readings, but if they are still abnormal despite an exercise program, they are still a risk. Remember, avid runners/athletes are not automatically protected from heart disease. Any uncontrolled risk factors are still problematic even in fit individuals — they can still act as pins to burst the endothelium lining and cause a heart attack or the slow accumulation of plaque. You have to protect yourself on *all* fronts.

Take you higher

Raise your HDL level by –
- Exercising
- Eating right
- Losing weight
- Not smoking
- Drinking moderately

A good diet helps

High fiber, low saturated fat, calorie balanced. High fiber, low saturated fat, calorie balanced. High fiber, low saturated fat, calorie balanced. (That's not a mistake — I meant to repeat these "ingredients" for emphasis). I'm going to harp on this again and again. We'll talk about diet in chapter 15. For now, it's important to remember that a healthy diet is absolutely vital to your heart-healthy existence and has far-reaching benefits, including a positive impact on your HDL cholesterol.

Weight off, HDL up

Appropriate weight loss will tend to improve HDL levels. Just as weight gain sets off the cycle of increased insulin and insulin resistance (shifting cholesterol production to the storage form of LDL), losing weight reverses these effects and more HDL (the non-storage form) tends to be produced. If you are overweight, losing weight will not only cause your joints and back to thank you, but will also result in a more favorable cholesterol profile and a happier heart.

Don't smoke

Quitting smoking raises HDL levels. If there weren't enough other reasons to stop, it appears that quitting smoking can result in a 15 to 20 percent increase in HDL levels . That's as good as what you'd expect from the best drugs available to raise HDL.

Drink moderately

Alcohol consumption, in moderate amounts, raises HDL. As I've already discussed in the chapter on heart failure, alcohol is a double-edged sword and one must strike the proper balance of consumption and health benefits. Consumed in excess, alcohol can become a destructive villain — physically, psychologically and socially — *and so I cannot and will not advise you to start drinking alcohol if you don't already drink; and I will not advise you to continue drinking if you have ever had any issues with excessive or inappropriate alcohol consumption.* However, for those of you who drink occasionally or moderately, continuing on with your practice is fine and may have long-term health benefits.

Again, moderate alcohol consumption is defined as one to two alcohol-containing drinks per day: one for women or smaller adults, two for men. One drink is defined as 12 ounces of beer, 5 ounces of wine, or 1 1/2 ounces of spirits (hard liquor such as gin or whiskey).

Studies suggest that *any* alcoholic beverage has beneficial effects when equivalent in alcohol content to the moderate definition. I would argue, however, that there's a tremendous difference between drinking a piña colada and a glass of merlot. Even moderate alcohol consumption can lose any potential benefit if various additives and mixes come along for the ride. The extra calories and sugars in the piña colada will annihilate any benefits of the alcohol content. So if you're choosing an alcoholic beverage, choose one that is least modified by mixes or other enhancements.

There may be additional benefits from drinking wine specifically, especially if it is dry and if it is red. Dry wine is relatively low in carbohydrates; red wine has a relatively high content of flavonoids (compounds with antioxidant properties).

> *To raise your HDL, eat right, exercise daily, attain or maintain a normal weight, stop smoking and, if appropriate for you, consume moderate amounts of alcohol.*

Despite all these efforts you might not see much of a change in your HDL number.

But don't be discouraged; there are a couple of things to keep in mind. First, HDL changes tend to be small (a five-point increase is considered a big deal). Second, even small differences in HDL translate into big benefits.

A 1 mg/dL increase in HDL translates into as much as a 6 percent decrease in cardiovascular risk. And even if you see little to no change in HDL levels, all the lifestyle changes you have made will translate into a healthier you.

OK, so far we've covered the good. Now let's talk about the bad.

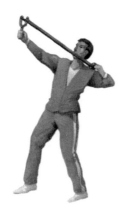

CHAPTER 8

The Bad—LDL

My doctor told me to stop having intimate dinners for four.
Unless there are three other people.
— Orson Welles (1915–1985)

L DL (low-density lipoprotein) is the bad cholesterol. LDL is the Lousy cholesterol and you want that number as **L**ow as possible. If HDL particles are the garbage trucks, LDL particles are the bags of garbage piling up in the streets.

This is the cholesterol that gums up your arteries and causes the buildup of blockages. LDL is the storage form of cholesterol. This is the cholesterol favored for deposition when insulin levels rise. It's also the cholesterol that is toxic to the lining of your arteries (that endothelium we talked about earlier). You can think of LDL as really sharp pins that increase the risk of a heart attack and/or stroke. It's not surprising then that LDL cholesterol most often becomes the target for treatment in patients with coronary artery disease (CAD) or those patients at high risk for developing CAD.

It can't go too low

The ideal levels of LDL cholesterol have been progressively ratcheted downward over the years. When I was training to be a cardiologist, an LDL level at or below 160 mg/dL was considered acceptable for everyone. In fact, I remember a significant concern amongst my mentors regarding the possible dangers of pushing LDL cholesterol levels below 120 mg/dL. Fifteen years later, no LDL cholesterol level is too low!

National scientific and medical organizations have outlined recommendations regarding optimal LDL levels. The guidelines state that an LDL of 160 mg/dL is the absolute upper limit of acceptable in patients without *any other risks* for heart disease. A level of 130 mg/dL or below is acceptable for individuals with some risk factors but no clinical evidence of heart problems (i.e., no history of previous heart attack, stroke, angioplasty, and so forth). Once you have had one of those events (i.e., you have documented heart disease), your LDL cholesterol should fall well below 100 mg/dL.

I would tell you that an LDL of 160 mg/dL makes most cardiologists shudder and that we are moving to officially lowering the goals for each group by 30 points. Most cardiologists would probably agree that 130 mg/dL is the upper limit of normal in most individuals without any other risk factors. As we accumulate risk factors (older age, high blood pressure, family history of heart disease, or tobacco use), the LDL level should optimally fall closer to or below 100 mg/dL. Once heart disease is known to be present, or there is evidence of vascular disease elsewhere, a history of stroke, or the patient has diabetes, the LDL cholesterol level should fall below 70 mg/dL. Achieving an LDL level below 70 mg/dL is very difficult if you depend on lifestyle changes alone; it usually requires the use of cholesterol-lowering medications.

Studies have shown that plaque buildup actually regresses in individuals being treated to lower their LDL levels below 70 mg/dL. The results are not miraculous; that is, you won't go from a 90 percent blockage to 0 percent, but it is possible to go from 90 percent to 60 percent. And even though plaque regression is not a complete cure, you can see how this small change could have a tremendous impact, knowing what you know about heart artery physiology and lanes on that superhighway. The buildup of gunk is a bit like putting straws on a camel's back. Eventually, you will put on one straw too many and the camel will fall down. Take that one straw away, and it can stand back up — at that critical point, small changes make a big difference.

Doctors and researchers have also noticed that patients who achieve very low LDL levels have significantly fewer heart attacks, even if there is little change in the severity of their blockages. This is where the endothelium and those balloons and pins and pothole analogies come back. You can think of a very low LDL as promoting pothole repair.

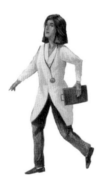

LDL Basics

Current published recommendations: (at the very least your numbers should reflect these)	
Minimum goal for everyone	below 160 mg/dL
Minimum goal if you have risk factors*	below 130 mg/dL
Minimum goal if you have coronary disease or coronary disease equivalent**	below 100 mg/dL
Get help!	over 160 mg/dL

More aggressive goals: (the goals more and more cardiologists recommend)	
Minimum goal for everyone	below 130 mg/dL
Minimum goal if you have risk factors*	below 100 mg/dL
Minimum goal if you have coronary disease or coronary disease equivalent**	below 70 mg/dL
Get help!	over 130 mg/dL

These include two or more of the following:

- *History of or current smoking*
- *High blood pressure*
- *Family history of heart disease*
- *Postmenopausal status (natural or due to surgical removal of the ovaries)*
- *Age over 50 for men and over 60 for women*

**These include any one or more of the following:*

- *Diabetes (even if not on any medications or insulin)*
- *History of stroke (even if minor or completely recovered from)*
- *Known blockages/atherosclerosis in any artery in the body (even if very minor)*

Down with LDL

How can you lower your LDL cholesterol? By following the exact same advice I gave for raising your HDL cholesterol. It turns out that a healthy lifestyle has healthy effects on your cholesterol profile, regardless of the cholesterol particle we're talking about. So following a healthy diet, getting regular exercise, and attaining and maintaining a good weight all contribute to lowering your LDL.

Smoking has little effect on LDL numbers per se. However, the products in tobacco smoke encourage the formation of oxidized LDL, a much more toxic form that is much more readily deposited in the arteries. Another reason to quit!

Alcohol intake appears to have little effect on LDL levels, and may even increase them due to the sugars contained in alcohol, which stimulate insulin release. (That's one of the reasons why the piña colada is clearly an inferior choice to the glass of merlot, and why more of a good thing is not always good.)

LDL levels can change dramatically with lifestyle changes. You can see 30- or 40-point drops — especially if your lifestyle is particularly unhealthy to begin with. So changes in LDL can be significantly more dramatic than the changes you see with HDL.

Occasionally I see patients whose LDL cholesterol level refuses to budge, despite their pristine existence. This tends to be a genetic effect. However, even if you can't make your numbers look better, you are much healthier for trying and should keep up the healthy lifestyle changes you have made.

LDL levels that start very high — well over 160 — tend to be genetically determined. Although adherence to a healthy lifestyle is still critical for these individuals, many (if not most) will end up on cholesterol-lowering medications to attain goal LDL levels.

Medications for lowering LDL are plentiful and effective. From a treatment perspective, of the three cholesterol particles that make up the cholesterol profile, LDL is the easiest to control with medications. Nevertheless, these medications are not a substitute for good eating habits or healthy lifestyle choices. Medications will also be much more effective (meaning you will need lower doses) if you do your part and live healthfully. Remember, all medications have potential side effects. Ideally, you want to live your life so you never need them. If you do require pills, you want to live your life so that you need as few medications — and at the smallest doses — as possible.

The rise in cholesterol that accompanies age translates principally into increases in LDL cholesterol. Postmenopausal women tend to see not only a fall in their HDL cholesterol but also a rise in LDL cholesterol. Checking your cholesterol profile regularly as you get older (and especially following menopause for women) is essential for making sure everything remains on track as far as your heart's health is concerned.

It's all relative

Sometimes it is confusing to understand the relationship between HDL and LDL levels, especially when both are high or both are low. For example, if the LDL is 90 mg/dL but the HDL is 30 mg/dL, which "wins" — the nice LDL number or the worrisome HDL number? Or what if the HDL is 80 mg/dL but the LDL is 168 mg/dL? Does the extra protection of the high HDL trump the you-should-be-on-medications LDL level?

For many years we have used something called the **cholesterol ratio** to help answer these questions. The cholesterol ratio basically attempts to determine whether enough of your garbage is being taken away to result in clean-enough streets.

The classic patient in whom the cholesterol ratio is examined is a woman with both high HDL and high LDL.

The cholesterol ratio is defined by the following formula:

> Cholesterol ratio = total cholesterol divided by HDL
> (ideal levels are less than 4)

Notice we're just concentrating on HDL and total cholesterol, even though the total is made up of several different numbers, including the TG level. Since HDL is the only "good" particle, we're looking at how much "good" there is relative to the total — both "good" and any "bad." Given the examples above, if a person's total cholesterol is 180 mg/dL (with an HDL level of 30 mg/dL), the ratio would be 180 divided by 30 or 6 — way too high. This means that the low LDL doesn't even come close to making up for the anemic HDL value. In the second example, if the total cholesterol is 280 mg/dL and the HDL level is 80 mg/dL, the ratio would be 280 divided by 80 or 3.5 — acceptable. Presumably the high LDL level is somewhat less worrisome in the second scenario.

In my own practice experience, I have found that the cholesterol ratio has limited utility. For the most part, I consider LDL and HDL as separate risk factors, and I attempt to optimize both values.

CHAPTER 9

And the Ugly — Triglycerides

I went into a McDonald's yesterday
and said, "I'd like some fries."
The girl at the counter said,
"Would you like some fries with that?"

— JAY LENO

Finally we come to **triglycerides (TGs)**. These are the ugly, not because they are more dangerous than LDL particles, but because when you take a sample of blood containing a lot of TGs (especially when TG levels are in the thousands) and let the sample sit in a test tube for a while, a separate layer of fat forms on the top (like cream floating to the top of a glass of very fatty milk). It's an ugly sight indeed!

Pancreatic impact

TG particles are different than the other two cholesterol particles. Triglycerides are one of the particles that transport fat around the body. Only about 20 percent of a TG particle consists of cholesterol. And the relative contribution of TGs to the development of heart disease has been less clear, compared to the definite roles of LDL and HDL.

Very high levels of TGs — over 400 mg/dL and especially over 1000 mg/dL — are associated with an increased risk of **pancreatitis** (inflammation of the pancreas). The pancreas is an organ that makes insulin as well as many enzymes that help digest food. When we eat, the pancreas (which is attached to the small intestine) dumps digestive enzymes through a series of channels into the lumen of the intestine to help break down foods.

When the pancreas becomes inflamed, the walls of the channels swell, blocking the exit of the digestive enzymes. The pancreas then, in essence, begins to digest itself, an extremely painful process that results in the scarring of the organ. Therefore, for patients with high triglyceride levels, medication may be prescribed to lower TG levels, not so much to prevent heart disease but to prevent pancreatitis.

Normal TG levels fall below 150 mg/dL.

Triglyceride Basics

Current published recommendations:	
Ideal for everyone	below 150 mg/dL
Worry about metabolic syndrome	over 150 mg/dL
Get help!	over 400 mg/dL

Worrisome profile

When TG levels are between 150 and 400 mg/dL, their significance depends on the company they keep rather than on their absolute values. In general, TG levels tend to mirror HDL levels in the opposite direction — patients with high HDL levels tend to have low TG levels and patients with low HDL levels tend to have high TG values. Obviously what you want is a high HDL and low TGs. The combination of low HDL and high TGs has recently been recognized as a particularly worrisome profile and has even been given its own name — **metabolic syndrome**.

Metabolic syndrome is most commonly seen in overweight or diabetic patients. It is also more likely in patients with truncal obesity (fat deposited around the waistline and chest, rather than in the hips) and those who are physically inactive. Patients with metabolic syndrome typically have high blood pressure.

Metabolic syndrome has been shown to have an even worse outcome than very high LDL levels.

Indeed, patients with metabolic syndrome are at especially high risk for developing heart disease, regardless of their LDL levels.

If your HDL level falls below 40 mg/dL and your TG level falls above 150 mg/dL, you may have metabolic syndrome and you need to do *everything* you can to change this situation. The metabolic syndrome is the ugliest of the ugly.

OK, that was the bad news. The good news about the ugly is that elevated triglycerides and even the metabolic syndrome pattern are exquisitely sensitive to lifestyle changes. Weight loss, dietary modification, and exercise can totally normalize cholesterol levels in these circumstances, and actually eliminate the metabolic syndrome pattern. The lifestyle alterations needed aren't necessarily minor, but desirable results are achievable without medications. However, I cannot emphasize this enough — *if you have metabolic syndrome, you must act now to correct it!*

Triglycerides are the most variable of the cholesterol numbers in the cholesterol profile. They also tend to play the role of the canary in the coal mine. They are often one of the first indicators that not all is well with your lifestyle choices. In fact, your doctor can often use the triglyceride levels to determine whether you've actually been staying on the straight and narrow. (We doctors can be sneaky!)

The TG twist

How can you lower your triglycerides? It's the old familiar recipe of good diet, exercise, and weight loss again — but with a couple of twists. Diet is especially powerful in influencing triglyceride levels. But not a low-fat diet. This might seem counterintuitive. (After all, TGs are primarily fat particles — right?) Yes, TGs are primarily fat particles, but they actually reflect an overabundance of carbohydrates rather than of actual fat in the diet.

Except in the situation where TG levels are extremely high (which tends to be genetically determined), TGs are around because they are efficient energy-storage particles. Our bodies clearly need some carbohydrates readily available for energy production, but we do not store all carbohydrates as carbohydrates; this would be very inefficient. Taking extra carbohydrates and turning them into TGs (essentially condensing them) makes storage much more compact. So anytime we have excess carbohydrates or higher (storage-promoting) insulin levels, TG levels tend to go up. You can therefore see how a low-fat diet (which is almost always high in carbohydrates) would be counterproductive in this situation.

The answer is a low-saturated-fat, high-fiber, calorie-controlled diet. Sound familiar? Just remember that *low saturated fat does not mean low fat.* A diet that includes **low saturated fat** encourages consumption of olive oil, canola oil, and the oils in nuts and seeds and fish. Low-carbohydrate diets actually work well in patients with high triglycerides, but for optimal health, a person must limit his or her consumption of saturated fats. High-saturated-fat intake is an often-overlooked side effect of many low-carb diets. (More on this in the chapter on diet.)

TG levels seem quite sensitive to weight loss also. I have noticed in my own patients that weight loss tends to result in a stepwise rather than gradual decrease in triglyceride levels. It's almost as if you need to prove your ability to shed a certain number of pounds before your body will reward you with a change in your TGs. The actual number of pounds required varies from person to person, so following your weight and your cholesterol numbers can be a bit of a frustrating process. But it also underscores the need to keep going with weight reduction until you get to your healthy weight; the full, positive cholesterol effects may not be evident until that point.

Change in the hundreds

Changes in triglyceride levels can be dramatic from an absolute numbers standpoint. Whereas we deal with single-digit changes for HDL cholesterol and low double-digit changes for LDL, TG changes can often be measured in the 100s (especially when you start out with a very high number). Amazingly, such changes can be seen with lifestyle management alone. Nothing underscores the benefits of a healthy existence like the sound of one of your bad cholesterol components dropping like a brick!

•

So now you have learned about the three main cholesterol numbers, what they mean and what influences their levels.

When and how often should you have these numbers checked? I think every adult should have their cholesterol profile checked once or twice in their 20s, with three checks in the 30s, four checks in the 40s, and yearly after age 50. This assumes acceptable levels and no major changes in health status, weight and so forth — otherwise you'll need more frequent evaluations. If you have a family history of very early coronary disease (e.g., your father had a heart attack in his early 50s), a history of marked cholesterol abnormalities in blood relatives, or a personal history of diabetes, start your cholesterol checks earlier and know that you may need to have them more frequently.

If you're over 30 and you've never had your cholesterol checked — what are you waiting for? Now is the time to take control of your health and your heart's destiny! Know your numbers. Know what they mean. Make all the changes you can to improve those numbers. Work with your doctor to develop a rational plan to prevent heart disease in yourself and energize your relatives and friends to do likewise.

Cholesterol capsule

Here's a quick reference summary of the major points from the past three chapters on cholesterol. Use this as a regular refresher, especially after you have gotten your cholesterol numbers checked.

- A **standard cholesterol profile** contains the total cholesterol and the three main particles that make up that total. These are HDL, LDL and triglycerides.
- The **total cholesterol number** is the least useful statistic from this whole profile, so if you want one less thing to remember, forget the total cholesterol.
- On the other hand, knowing your **HDL, LDL and TG levels** is vital to being an active and informed participant in your personal crusade to ward off heart disease.
- **HDL** particles can be thought of as garbage trucks. These cholesterol particles are on their way to being removed, and you want this number as high as possible.
- **LDL** particles are like bags of garbage that pile up and gum up your arteries. You want this number to be as low as possible.
- **Triglycerides (TGs)** are a health risk when very high on their own (especially >1000 mg/dL) because of the increased risk of pancreatitis. Triglyceride elevation as an isolated finding contributes to heart disease risk but less so than HDL or LDL levels.
- The combination of low HDL and high triglycerides is a particularly toxic one and is referred to as **metabolic syndrome**, which puts the patient at an especially high risk for developing heart disease over time.
- All **cholesterol abnormalities** tend to improve with healthy lifestyle changes. Triglycerides are most sensitive to lifestyle changes, while HDL is least sensitive.
- Start **measuring your cholesterol profile** in your 20s — at the very least by 30. The frequency of subsequent measurements depends upon the findings and your overall health status. Discuss your particular situation with your doctor to come up with a reasonable monitoring plan.

Piece of Advice #4

Know your cholesterol profile, know your numbers, get involved and get active. Keep on task to get your numbers checked regularly and be sure they fall in the desirable range for your particular situation. *You* are in control of your cardiovascular destiny. Sit on the sidelines too long and your career may end prematurely.

Visit <u>www.CardioSmart.org</u> for tools and information to help you track and manage your cholesterol profile

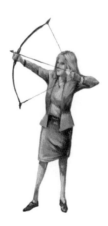

CHAPTER 10

Beyond the Regular Cholesterol Profile

Health nuts are going to feel stupid someday,
lying in hospitals dying of nothing.
— REDD FOXX (1922–1991)

O K — I've got you thinking about HDL and LDL and metabolic syndrome. This is a great beginning and hopefully you're motivated to look up your numbers or get them checked. In this chapter, I'm going to talk about some other blood tests that could further define your risk. Not all of these tests are appropriate for everyone, so I will try to point out which type of patient benefits from having which additional tests.

A word of caution: Not all of these tests are recognized by all physicians as useful or necessary, so even if by my estimation you fit the criteria of someone who might benefit from these tests, your health-care provider might think differently. If nothing else, it's worth a conversation. There are no absolutes here — knowledge in this area is evolving. After you read this chapter, you will one day undoubtedly run across news articles and studies that disagree with what I've written, and shortly thereafter find other reports that vehemently support the advice you'll find here.

I tend to err on the side of "overprevention" rather than "underprevention." And as long as the testing is relatively straightforward and the treatment required is not otherwise harmful, causes side effects, or is overly complex, I do what I can to normalize or at least neutralize potential risk factors in the patients I see.

Let's start with LDL.

A fraction of a fraction

But, wait, you say — didn't we already do LDL? Well, yes we did. But I didn't explain earlier that the LDL cholesterol number does not provide you with all the information about your LDL that you might need.

Your LDL number (as you probably noticed in the previous chapter) is usually provided as a value that is in **mg/dL** — or milligrams per deciliter. Huh?? A **milligram** is a unit of weight and a **deciliter** is a unit of volume. So your LDL value in milligrams per deciliter tells you that you have a certain weight of LDL cholesterol in a certain volume of blood. This actually discloses nothing about the *number* of LDL particles circulating in your blood stream. The total weight might be made up of a few large particles or many small particles — small particles being worse, since they can more easily sneak into artery walls and in any total LDL number there would be more of them. Under ideal circumstances you want to have a **L**ow LDL number made up of **L**arge LDL particles.

You would think that knowing the actual LDL particle number (or at least particle size) might be a much more important piece of information than knowing your LDL mg/dL amount (and it probably is). But it turns out that this information is much more difficult to obtain, generally requiring a rather expensive test that is available only through certain specialized laboratories. We do have some clues about LDL particle size based upon other findings in the cholesterol profile — for example, patients with metabolic syndrome tend to have small LDL particles (a double whammy!) — making it less critical to check this test in some patients.

Analyze this

Furthermore, most of the major studies that have looked at the effects of cholesterol on heart disease have dealt with the mg/dL-type LDL measurements, and all the recommendations for LDL goals have used the mg/dL values, removing LDL particle number and size from routine clinical use. So if your doctor has never checked your LDL particle number (or size), you are not alone. This test is called **LDL sub fraction analysis** and is used in very select circumstances only. I'll get to which circumstances a little later in this chapter.

Now let's talk about HDL. It turns out that what's true for LDL is also true for HDL. HDL can exist in different forms and large HDL particles are more efficient garbage trucks than small HDL particles. You want **H**igh numbers of **H**uge HDL particles. So even if you have a normal HDL level according to the mg/dL analysis, it may not be as protective as you think if the HDL is in the wrong form.

The same specialized laboratories that perform LDL sub fraction analysis also perform **HDL sub fraction analysis**, and these tests are usually ordered together.

Regular exercise, a healthy diet and the attainment and maintenance of a healthy weight tend to favor the presence of big (and more favorable) HDL and LDL particles.

How many times am I going to say the same thing about diet, exercise and weight control? Hundreds! Get used to it!

When a little is a lot

We can also measure the **lipoprotein A** particle (**Lp(a)**, sometimes referred to quite scientifically as "L-P-little-a"). Lp(a) is an LDL cholesterol particle with an extra protein attached to it. This slight modification is in fact a big deal, making the LDL more toxic and expanding the amount of chaos it can create. Lp(a) appears to contribute to higher clotting propensity — which, given what you now know about heart attacks and strokes, is clearly not ideal.

The lipoprotein A level is hidden in the LDL measurement, and unless you assess it specifically, you can't tell how much of the LDL is in Lp(a) form.

Normal levels of Lp(a) generally fall under 30 mg/dL.

The upper limits of normal can vary from laboratory to laboratory; keep this variability in mind. Lp(a) appears to be genetically determined and really can't be changed much by lifestyle or medications. Some variability exists in the measurement from one time to the next, but the values tend to remain in the same general range over time. This is a test you need only once or twice in your life (certainly *not* every time you get your cholesterol profile checked).

Stuck on you

Homocysteine (ho-mo-CIS-teen) is another blood test. Homocysteine is not a cholesterol particle and does not deposit in your arteries. Rather, it makes the artery walls "stickier" — more likely to grab on to any cholesterol that's around.

Homocysteine is a by product of protein metabolism, and genetics and B-vitamin levels influence its levels. Changing your diet by reducing protein intake will usually not have a major impact on homocysteine, however.

Normal homocysteine levels usually fall well below 15 mg/dL.

Again, normal values can differ from lab to lab. Folic acid (folate), vitamins B6 and B12 all lower homocysteine levels — therefore getting an adequate supply of these nutrients is important. Homocysteine levels in the general population have fallen over time because more and more foods are supplemented with folate and B vitamins. In addition to advising patients to consume healthy foods, I usually advise my patients to take a daily multivitamin regardless of baseline homocysteine level, just to make sure that they get plenty of B vitamins. I do not prescribe specific vitamin B supplements routinely.

Out with inflammatory

C-reactive protein (cRP) is a blood test that measures the level of inflammation in our bodies. Inflammation occurs when tissues of the body respond to injury or irritation; **inflammatory cells** (specialized blood cells that circulate in our bloodstreams and deposit in areas of injury) mediate this response. Inflammation can manifest itself as swelling, redness or pain. The reaction of the skin to a mosquito bite is a good example (those of us living in Minnesota have LOTS of experience with this!). Although inflammation can be a component of an infection, inflammation is *not* the same as infection.

It turns out that part of the atherosclerotic process — the process of laying down gunk in our arteries — is inflammatory. If you look at an artery wall under the microscope, you will see inflammatory cells along with the cholesterol particles. Among other things, inflammatory cells cause the release of cRP.

It's been noted that groups of patients with elevated cRP levels have a higher risk of developing heart attacks or strokes, compared to patients with low levels of cRP. The reason may be that when there is more C-reactive protein there are more inflammatory cells within the walls of the arteries, and the atherosclerotic process is more active. If the process of laying down the gunk is more active, the plaque itself is in the process of change, and is therefore less stable and more prone to breaking down. And if you recall from our original discussions, unstable plaque and endothelial disruption can lead to heart attacks and strokes. So a high cRP level may actually be a marker of endothelial vulnerability.

These observations and explanations work well when looking at groups of patients (which is how most medical trials are done). It's less straightforward when dealing with separate individuals, since cRP is not a very specific marker; inflammatory cells anywhere in the body can cause cRP levels to rise. Also, the laying down of gunk in our arteries ebbs and flows, and does not occur at a steady rate. Thus, cRP levels can vary from time to time.

So an elevated cRP level may not always indicate a problem with the coronary arteries, and a normal cRP level isn't totally reassuring. It's easy, therefore, to see why the cardiology community are still split about the true value of this test. Nevertheless, more and more compelling data is emerging regarding cRP and the degree to which different levels identify patients with different cardiovascular destinies.

> *The normal level of cRP is considered below 1 mg/dL, and for treatment purposes, a desirable level is below 2 mg/ dL.*

Cholesterol in hiding

Other blood tests can be done to help define heart disease risk. Occasionally we identify patients with high **VLDL** or **IDL** levels (**very-low-density-** and **intermediate-density lipoprotein**, respectively). It turns out that, besides LDL, HDL and triglycerides, other types of cholesterol particles circulate in the bloodstream. Since we typically only measure the total cholesterol, TG and HDL cholesterol (and calculate the LDL), the remaining cholesterol particles tend to be hidden within that calculated LDL number. One way of acknowledging the existence of all these other cholesterol particles is to talk about **non-HDL cholesterol**.

> *Non-HDL cholesterol is defined as total cholesterol minus HDL. Ideally this should be under 130 mg/dL.*

Not another number or goal to remember! Actually, you already know this goal based on the information you've already learned and the numbers and goals you already know, as shown in the accompanying box.

Non-HDL Cholesterol

You know that:

$$\text{Total cholesterol} = \text{HDL} + \text{LDL} + (\text{TG/5})$$

Actually, that formula is more accurately represented as:

$$\text{Total cholesterol} =$$
$$\text{HDL} + (\text{LDL} + \text{other cholesterol particles}) + (\text{TG/5})$$

I didn't give you this formula to begin with, because "other cholesterol particles" are rarely the sole reason for high total cholesterol levels, and because the last few chapters were overwhelming enough!

$$\text{Total cholesterol} - \text{HDL} =$$
$$(\text{LDL} + \text{other cholesterol particles}) + (\text{TG/5})$$

In other words:

$$\text{Non-HDL cholesterol} =$$
$$(\text{LDL} + \text{other cholesterol particles}) + (\text{TG/5})$$

Non-HDL cholesterol should be below 130 mg/dL because TGs should ideally be below 150 mg/dL (this number divided by five should amount to under 30 points) and because the sum of LDL and the other particles in the perfect universe would always fall below 100 mg/dL. In some ways, the non-HDL cholesterol measurement is akin to the cholesterol ratio — again we're dealing only with the total number and the HDL number in the calculation. Most cardiologists currently consider the non-HDL number to be more clinically useful than the cholesterol ratio, and more likely to identify patients at risk.

Boutique shopping

Finally, there are several "boutique" tests. These range from tests determining insulin levels to those detecting protein markers on cholesterol particles to those looking at blood clotting/dissolving factors. There are many others. I will not discuss these, since they are either applicable to a very small number of people, are not easily available or are investigational at this time. The bottom line? Defining risk using **serologic markers** (analyzing substances within blood) is an active area of research and more and better defined markers will probably emerge. It's always a good idea to ask your doctor from time to time if any new tests to assess risk are available, and if they would be useful in your particular case.

Several researchers are investigating the degree to which infectious agents, like certain viruses and bacteria, contribute to the formation of plaque. So far the research has been inconclusive, and the use of antibiotics to "cure" or "prevent" heart disease is not recommended. Although the chances that an underlying infection is the reason for plaque formation seem slim, it's probably still prudent to keep your eyes open for studies coming out on this topic. I learned a long time ago to never say never in the world of medicine.

Piece of Advice #5

When you visit with your doctor, especially in the context of a general or yearly exam, always ask if there are any new tests for better defining your risk of heart or blood vessel disease — or that screen for any other diseases that you may be at risk for developing. You have to be proactive and look out for your own interests. Prompting your physician is not rude or pushy — it's your body and it's your life. If there is a test that could affect your body or your life, asking about its availability and application to your situation only makes sense.

Which ones when?

I said earlier that the additional tests are worth doing under certain circumstances. What are those circumstances?

Patients with a family history of heart disease (especially if one or more blood relatives have experienced coronary disease or stroke at a young age) and **patients with more advanced heart disease than expected for their age** would benefit from having most of these additional tests run. Repeated testing would need to be considered depending on the initial results.

Lipoprotein A and particle size. Particle size analys is (LDL and HDL sub fraction evaluation), being relatively expensive tests, could be reserved for the specific circumstance of a relatively normal cholesterol profile (with normal Lp(a), homocysteine and cRP) in the setting of a family or personal history of accelerated atherosclerosis. In most other situations we can make most prevention decisions based upon analyzing the regular cholesterol profile in conjunction with any other risk factors that may be present.

A patient with an unfavorable cholesterol particle size or increased Lp(a) would need to have his or her goal LDL lowered by one category — so if your goal LDL was 100 based upon other factors and your Lp(a) came back at 67 mg/dL, I would favor trying to push your LDL to well below 70 mg/dL. If your LDL goal was 130 mg/dL, but all your LDL particles were small, I would want to see your LDL well below 100 mg/dL. Basically, an abnormality of particle size or Lp(a) raises the stakes for preventive efforts: *You* need to double your efforts toward diet, exercise and weight control, and *your doctor* may need to recommend cholesterol-lowering medications earlier.

Lipoprotein A levels tend to remain stable over time regardless of what you or your doctor does. Although some studies have shown that Lp(a) levels can be reduced with high-dose niacin therapy (niacin is a vitamin, but the doses used in treatment are so high that it essentially needs to be thought of as a drug), I've found (as have many other cardiologists) that the impact of niacin on Lp(a) levels is minor — and that any improvement seen with treatment is probably due to the natural variation that can occur with Lp(a) measurements.

Over time I have abandoned the use of niacin as the primary method of treating an elevated Lp(a). My current strategy (and that of many cardiologists) is to go after the LDL rather than the Lp(a) — to lower the LDL level *way down*, at least 30 points lower than the number that a doctor might recommend based upon the other risk factors. The logic behind this strategy is this: If Lp(a) makes LDL particles more toxic in general and we can't get rid of the Lp(a) very easily, we should try to minimize the number of LDL particles floating around — so that even if they're more toxic than normal, at least there aren't very many of them. If the goal LDL starts at 70 mg/dL or below, aiming for 40 mg/dL is probably not realistic. But being stringent about keeping the LDL below 70 mg/dL is essential.

I think Lp(a) should be checked at least once for *everyone* regardless of other risks. If you're starting to check your regular cholesterol profile in your 30s, having a Lp(a) analysis done at the same time is reasonable. If the level is fine, probably rechecking it again in your 50s is reasonable. If the level is abnormal, the abnormality should be confirmed with a repeat test and you should jump into preventive action ASAP. You might not need medications, but really getting serious and consistent with a healthy lifestyle will prove critical.

Homocysteine. If you have a personal or family history of accelerated atherosclerosis, you should have your homocysteine checked. If your levels are in the normal range, rechecking your homocysteine level is probably not required unless there are major changes in your health status. (There are no clear guidelines for this — this recommendation is based solely on my opinion and practice experience.)

If your homocysteine levels are elevated, you may need some additional blood work — including blood tests to check thyroid function, and vitamin B6, B12 and folate levels. Occasionally, even more blood work is required to confidently rule in or rule out a vitamin deficiency. Currently, treatment of elevated homocysteine levels consists of vitamin supplementation

— especially with folate. Amounts of folate required to normalize homocysteine levels are variable, and occasionally very high doses are required (5 mg or more, compared to the typical multivitamin that contains less than 500 µg — 1/10th of this amount), but virtually every patient responds to treatment eventually.

Although treatment can normalize homocysteine levels, it is not clear whether improvement in those levels translates into reduced risk of heart disease over time. In my mind, it seems reasonable to reduce or normalize homocysteine levels in those patients with evidence of early coronary disease or a strong family history of CAD. Certainly, the treatment is safe and inexpensive, so I tend to hedge on the side of treating abnormal homocysteine levels in this patient subset.

You should be aware that an elevated homocysteine level may be a marker of some other underlying health issue (such as low thyroid function, kidney disease or B-vitamin deficiency) that warrants treatment in its own right. With adequate treatment of these disorders, homocysteine levels can normalize as a secondary benefit.

C-reactive protein (cRP). It is not clear how to use cRP levels in patients who have no known coronary disease. *If you already have CAD,* you should probably have your cRP level checked, and you should aim to normalize that level (get it at least below 2 mg/L). This might necessitate increasing your cholesterol-lowering medications even further than would be considered adequate if determined by your LDL alone.

If you don't have known CAD, I'm not sure that random cRP tests are appropriate. I think it might make sense for you to check your cRP level once you have brought all of your markers under appropriate control for your particular situation. At that point, evaluating your cRP as a last check would be reasonable so that you could see whether your treatment regimen is adequate for your arteries.

Another situation in which I might check cRP is one involving patients with a personal or family history of accelerated atherosclerosis, who also have relatively normal cholesterol profiles (the same patients I'd be thinking about checking a HDL/LDL cholesterol sub fraction analysis in). I would also consider checking cRP in patients with conflicting test results in terms of risk (high HDL, high LDL, for example) or patients with borderline indications for starting medications to control one or more risk factors.

Basically, in patients without known CAD, I use the cRP as a tie-breaker or treatment validator.

Some physicians feel differently about this test, and might order it every time they check the cholesterol profile. This is one of those circumstances where our knowledge is evolving and new data might influence recommendations regarding cRP testing after this book has been published. I would advise you to talk to your personal physician and discuss whether he or she feels you might benefit from this test, given your particular circumstances and risk profile.

What can you do for an elevated cRP? Since a high level is a marker of inflammation, use of an anti-inflammatory medication (i.e., aspirin) makes sense, and most physicians will recommend taking a daily aspirin. Because the inflammation is presumably a response to more accelerated deposition of gunk in the arteries, minimizing all modifiable risk factors in the hope of stopping or slowing the atherosclerotic process will also be essential. So we're back to adopting an exemplary lifestyle of weight control, blood pressure control and the lowering of cholesterol (moving those cholesterol goals down 30 points for every LDL category). In some cases, you might attain your lowest LDL goals but will still not be able to normalize the cRP. Your doctor may increase your medications until the cRP is normalized, irrespective of how low the LDL goes (this would be expected to occur only rarely, however).

> *We're establishing a theme here. For these "other" blood markers that indicate risk, if abnormal, double up your lifestyle correction attempts, and understand that in some cases your LDL goal will need to be more stringent by at least one category (30 points lower than the goal would have been without one of these additional abnormal markers).*

Best by test

This chapter describes markers of heart disease risk that may, above and beyond a cholesterol profile, add additional information about your particular situation —

- These markers can be measured with blood tests, although specialized laboratories may need to perform the analyses and the tests may be expensive.

- All of these tests should be considered for patients with a personal or family history of early or accelerated heart disease.

- LDL and HDL sub fraction analysis should probably be reserved for those situations in which, despite other testing, the reason for an accelerated atherosclerotic process is unclear.

- Everyone should have their lipoprotein A levels checked at least once in their lives.

- Homocysteine testing should probably be reserved only for those patients with accelerated atherosclerosis or a strong family history of CAD.

- The story about C-reactive protein is evolving and this test may become more widely utilized for risk assessment as more data emerge. At the present time, it is reasonable to use this test as a double check on the completeness of prevention efforts.

- In general, if an abnormality of any of these additional markers exists, it is a signal that you need to kick your prevention efforts to higher gear — from crossing all the *t*'s and dotting all the *i*'s in your diet, exercise program and weight-control efforts, to tightening the goals for your cholesterol numbers.

Piece of Advice #6

If you have a strong family history of heart disease (especially
if you have relatives who have experienced heart attacks,
angioplasties, bypass surgeries or strokes at relatively young
ages), talk to your doctor about having some of these additional
tests run. These tests can point out risk factors that may be genetically
transmitted, but are not obvious from the regular cholesterol profile
evaluation. When it comes to prevention, you need to dot the *i*'s and
cross the *t*'s.

CHAPTER 11

It's a Pressure Cooker Out There!

In all our efforts to provide "advantages"
we have actually produced the busiest, most
competitive, highly pressured, and over-organized
generation...in our history.
— Eda J. Le Shan

We've just covered information about markers of heart disease risk that can be discovered by blood tests. Measuring blood pressure requires no needles — in fact, you can even check your own yourself. Now here's a risk factor you can take control of and monitor very easily! It can be completely controlled and any threat from it eliminated.

And yet, **hypertension** (high blood pressure) remains an under-diagnosed and under-treated risk factor. Currently, hypertension affects about 50 million people in our country and approximately 1 *billion* individuals worldwide. (Did I just hear you say WOW?) Furthermore,

more and more people engage in more and more behaviors that encourage hypertension — as we become more sedentary, heavier, and eat more and more processed and salt-rich foods, we set ourselves up for high blood pressure. The stress of our go-go-go world doesn't help. And we can't wipe out something we're not measuring or monitoring. Now is the time for you to get to know your blood pressure levels and what your goals should be, and to learn how you can reach those goals.

Consider the cuff

Two numbers make up your blood pressure — the **systolic** (CIS-tuh-lyk) blood pressure (the "top number") and the **diastolic** (DYE-ah-STO-lyk) blood pressure (the "bottom number"). So in a typical blood pressure reading of 130/80 mmHg, 130 is the systolic value and 80 is the diastolic reading.

When your doctor measures your blood pressure, he or she blows up the blood pressure cuff to a pressure above your systolic reading, and then slowly lets the air out of the cuff while listening over an artery on the inside of your arm. The pressure in the cuff eventually drops (reflected in the drop of a column of mercury within a calibrated tube — hence the recording of blood pressure in **mmHg,** or millimeters of mercury) below your systolic pressure. At that time, your doctor hears the pulsations of blood in your arm (and you might feel a pulsation in your hand or forearm). The first point at which this sound is heard is recorded as the systolic blood pressure. As the cuff pressure is released further, it eventually drops below your diastolic blood pressure, and at that point, the pulsations heard through the stethoscope become significantly muffled or disappear entirely. The pressure at which the pulsations first become muffled is recorded as the diastolic blood pressure.

> *A normal systolic blood pressure is considered at or below 120 mmHg, and a normal diastolic blood pressure is considered at or below 80 mmHg.*

Just like cholesterol goals, the goals for blood pressure readings have been getting more stringent. Many years ago, hypertension was defined as a blood pressure over 160/90 mmHg measured at rest on at least two separate occasions, and readings below that were considered generally acceptable. At the present time, the definition of hypertension has been reduced to a reading above 140/90 mmHg, and the higher reading of 160/90 mmHg is now considered "severe" or "grade 2" hypertension. A blood pressure over 120/80 mmHg but below 140/90 mmHg (measured at rest on at least two separate occasions) has come to define **prehypertension**, and a blood pressure at or below 120/80 mmHg has been defined as normal.

Blood pressures between 120/80 mmHg and 139/89 mmHg are considered worrisome enough that people with these readings should try to change aspects of their lifestyles that contribute to elevated blood pressures. Indeed, recent data suggest that patients with prehypertension have a threefold increase in their risk of having a heart attack.

Pulse pressure

Another blood pressure measurement can also infer increased risk — this is the pulse pressure. The pulse pressure is the numeric difference between your systolic and diastolic blood pressure. For example, if your resting blood pressure is 140/90 mmHg, your pulse pressure is 50 — the difference between 140 and 90. It turns out that a high pulse pressure can indicate the presence of stiff or damaged blood vessels. And if you have stiff or damaged blood vessels in your arms, you almost certainly have stiff or damaged blood vessels in your heart. The pulse pressure is especially important in patients older than 60 years of age. A pulse pressure over 60 is considered abnormal. Treating high blood pressure usually reduces pulse pressure as well.

In patients with diabetes or those with known cardiovascular or kidney disease, doctors currently recommend that resting blood pressures be maintained well below 130/85 mmHg. And even if patients' pressures initially fall within the upper prehypertension range, if their readings are not below 130/85 mmHg, they should use medications to get them there.

Why have the numbers used to define hypertension fallen? Over the years we have found that lower blood pressure is always better, and that there appears to be a progressive decrease in the chance of experiencing heart disease or stroke with falling BP levels. In patients with hypertension, medical treatment to lower blood pressures has been shown to reduce the risk of stroke by 35 to 40 percent, the risk of a heart attack by 20 to 25 percent, and the risk of heart failure by 50 percent. In patients with "mild" ("grade 1") hypertension (BP of 140–159/90–99 mmHg), reducing the systolic blood pressure by 10 mmHg for 10 years prevents one death for every 10 patients treated. That's an *amazing* reduction in risk for a small reduction in blood pressure readings. So it's not just about making your numbers look better — *treating high blood pressure is about saving lives.*

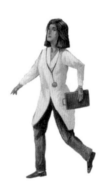

Pressure points

Hypertension is a major contributor to heart disease, and the *number one* preventable cause of heart failure.

- A normal blood pressure is defined as less than or equal to 120/80 mmHg. The systolic ("top number") reading is often used for assessment of blood pressure control.

- You should be concerned if you are seeing blood pressure readings over 130 mmHg systolic or 85 mmHg diastolic at your health checkups.

- Obesity, tobacco use, lack of exercise, high sodium consumption, and sleep apnea are all contributors to hypertension that can be modified or reversed.

- If your readings are not optimal, become an active participant. A home monitor is relatively inexpensive and can be extremely helpful.

- Know what your readings are and where you fit on the spectrum of blood pressure readings. Hypertension is a modifiable risk factor.

- Many medications can be used to lower blood pressure. At times it requires several attempts of different dosages and combinations of medications to attain the desired result.

- How you live your life, how you control your weight and what you eat can have a dramatic effect on your blood pressure control. Be proactive in your own care.

Underdiagnosed condition

Getting back to that statement I made earlier about how hypertension is under-diagnosed and undertreated ... Can you guess the percentage of hypertensive people in the United States who control their readings? (I'm not even talking about below 120/80 mmHg — I'm just talking about below 140/90 mmHg.) You'll never guess — 34 percent.

That means 66 percent — *two thirds* — of all people with hypertension are not adequately controlling their blood pressures. Aren't you astounded? Do you want to be more amazed? Thirty percent of the people with hypertension aren't *even aware* that they have a problem. For something so easy to monitor, we're sure missing the boat.

Untreated hypertension is one of the leading causes of heart failure. And just as the initial phases of heart failure can be completely silent, hypertension is completely silent also. So you could be literally destroying your heart without knowing it.

And here's the really scary part — even patients with early, often asymptomatic heart muscle stiffening related to hypertension (abnormal diastolic function) have markedly worse prognoses than those who don't. Bottom line is — *heart damage from hypertension can kill you regardless of the extent of underlying coronary disease,* because hypertension can take you down a one-way street toward heart failure.

There is a reason hypertension has been labeled "the silent killer." That's exactly what it is. It not only contributes to the development of atherosclerotic disease, it also is *the* major preventable cause of heart failure.

Essentially hypertensive

What causes hypertension? The vast majority of the time, hypertension has no one identifiable cause and is given the label "essential hypertension."

Even though the condition is "essential," however, lifestyle factors clearly contribute to the severity of blood pressure elevations. In fact, adherence to a healthy lifestyle can go a long way toward causing your readings to fall and avoiding the need for medications, or at least reducing the amount of medications required to control your BP readings.

There are other reasons why patients have high blood pressures, but these are quite uncommon and because they involve disorders in other organ systems, I will not enumerate or explain them here. If you have blood pressures that are difficult to control, or you experience a relatively sudden change in your blood pressure readings, your doctor may undertake further testing to see if any of these rare causes of hypertension are present. But most of the time, we (at least initially) assume the hypertension is "essential" because it almost always is.

Lifestyle factors that contribute to higher readings include being overweight, being sedentary, smoking, consuming excessive amounts of alcohol and taking in large amounts of sodium. Sounds a bit like the list of factors that cause coronary disease, doesn't it? I have to say it again — can't help myself — *healthy diet, regular exercise and weight reduction.* We're back to the cornerstones of staying healthy and warding off heart disease (and hypertension, too).

Obviously, if you **smoke**, you must quit, regardless of your blood pressure readings! Lowering your blood pressure readings will be only one of the myriad health benefits you will realize when you stop lighting up. The toxins in tobacco smoke cause **vasoconstriction** (narrowing or spasm of your blood vessels), and this directly causes your blood pressure to go up. After quitting smoking, vasoconstriction can quickly improve and blood pressures decline. This is just one of the reasons for the almost immediate reduction in risk when patients quit using tobacco.

You'll need to modify your **alcohol consumption** if you have hypertension. Finding the balance between benefit and harm becomes more difficult here, and some physicians will counsel patients to avoid alcoholic beverages altogether if they have hypertension. I'm a bit more lenient in this regard (probably because I enjoy a glass of wine myself). I advise my patients that continuing with *moderate* alcohol intake (no more than the equivalent of one to two glasses of wine per day, with the lower amount for women and smaller men) is acceptable unless we run into difficulties controlling blood pressure with medications or if the situation is borderline and the patient is on the verge of needing to start medications. Under either of those circumstances I suggest that alcohol be eliminated from the equation because I would like to nullify any possible culprit or contributor to blood pressure elevation.

Pounds, years, and sleep

Excess weight is a huge (pardon the pun) contributor to high blood pressure. The fatter you get, the more likely it is that your pressures will rise above normal levels. Most patients who are overweight have blood pressure readings that are not optimal and many require medications (especially with the newest guidelines and definitions). The good news is that, with normalization of body weight, blood pressures can come down significantly, reducing or eliminating the need for antihypertensive medications.

Blood pressures tend to go up with **age** and, unless you remain fairly physically active, metabolism goes down at the same time. Excess weight magnifies the effect of age on blood pressure readings. So if you are young and overweight, you must start a weight-loss campaign immediately. If you let your weight continue to stay elevated, or to increase further, you are walking into a trap — as time goes on, it will become harder and harder to lose the weight and your blood pressures will go up and up.

A condition that can accompany excess weight is **sleep apnea** (AP-nee-ya). Occasionally, people who are not overweight experience it. Sleep apnea is the condition in which sleep is repeatedly disrupted because of disturbed breathing patterns. Men with neck circumferences over 17 inches and women with neck circumferences over 16 inches are at increased risk for this disorder. Common symptoms of sleep apnea include marked or loud snoring, witnessed periods of apnea (breathing that has stopped) while asleep and excessive daytime sleeepiness. Sleep apnea contributes to hypertension and its successful treatment can result in significantly lower blood pressure readings. I have personally taken care of several patients whose blood pressures completely normalized once their sleep apnea symptoms were addressed. Sleep apnea can itself cause problems with heart muscle relaxation, causing diastolic dysfunction and, eventually, heart failure. This is not just an issue of loud snoring. It's a potentially life-limiting disease.

If you find that you repeatedly doze off during the day, feel persistently tired while awake, and/or have had others comment on your snoring or sleeping patterns, talk to your doctor. These symptoms might indicate the presence of underlying sleep apnea and several treatment options exist. Sleep apnea doesn't only affect blood pressure and therefore its treatment is not only reserved for patients with hypertension. Because this disorder has far-reaching effects, treatment should be sought even if the person with the sleep apnea has normal blood pressures.

No pain, no grain

People who are fit, in general, have lower resting heart rates and lower resting blood pressures than do people who are sedentary. If we exercise regularly, our bodies adapt by becoming more and more efficient, such that for any level of exertion, heart rate and blood pressure rise more slowly and remain lower than in unfit individuals. If you have hypertension or find yourself in the prehypertension category, getting active and staying active are *essential* components of getting and keeping your blood pressure down. Even if you do not have high blood pressures, getting active is important, since aging is against you and you want to hit your middle and later years as fit and healthy as possible.

Take a look at what you eat. Unless you cook all your own food, you have very little control over the sodium content of your food choices. And the decks are stacked against you. Over time, food manufacturers and preparers have figured out that sweeter and saltier food items tend to appeal more to consumers and therefore sell more. This has resulted in a subtle (or maybe not so subtle) shift over time toward progressively more sodium- and sugar-laden foods. Ironically, to get all the sodium we need in our diets for health, we don't need to add *any* salt to *any* food we eat or prepare. So every grain of salt added to our food is salt we don't need.

Now, I'm not going to advise you to never consume any salt ever again — this is not realistic, and let's face it, some salt does make certain foods taste better. But the amounts we use and consume must be reduced. Many of us will need to retrain our palates. And we will all need to start being more vigilant about the sodium content of foods. The best way to accomplish this is to start cooking all your own meals from scratch. Yeah, I know — as if! But being more involved in food preparation will help you to exert some control over what you take in. So try to cook at least some if not most of your food. And when you can't, become a label fiend and check out the sodium content of what you're eating.

When it comes to sodium content, the main culprits are heavily processed foods. Chips, snack mixes, fast foods and luncheon meats are often especially loaded with sodium — but seasoning mixes (e.g., taco seasoning), crackers, canned soups and vegetables, and many ready-prepared food items can be even worse than chips when it comes to sodium content. *The fresher and less complicated the item, the less likely it is to be loaded with salt.* Read labels! Control what's going into your body.

How much sodium should we be consuming? For sure under 2400 mg of sodium/day — that's the sodium content of one teaspoon of table salt. I'm talking about *your whole day's* consumption here — that one teaspoon has to last you the whole day. And you'd be surprised how quickly the sodium adds up. A slice of whole wheat bread has 140 mg, a cup of reduced-salt broth still has 570 mg, a taco salad has around 1000 mg!

Some people have blood pressures that are very salt sensitive, and others have blood pressures that are not influenced in the least by the sodium content of their diets. Many people fall somewhere in between. You won't know which camp you fall into until you try to reduce your sodium consumption and see where you land. It can take several weeks to see the effect, however, so don't judge your response too early. Regardless of your concerns about your blood pressure, reducing sodium in your diet is healthy in general because you will likely reduce the proportion of heavily processed or modified foods in your diet — which will result in a generally healthier eating plan. And after your sodium reduction experiment, I suspect you will find your previous dietary choices far too salty for your new palate.

Piece of Advice #7

Commit to examining your diet and analyze where most of your sodium intake comes from. This will almost certainly involve reading food labels and even requesting nutritional information in restaurants and at the supermarket. And remember your goal: less than 2400 milligrams of sodium per day.

Piece of Advice #8

Experiment with reducing sodium content in your diet. You can make gradual changes (e.g., not adding any salt to prepared foods) or dramatic changes (e.g., preparing all your own meals from scratch). Although the latter is ideal, I think aiming for at least a mixture of the two extremes is realistic for all of us. Follow your reduced-sodium approach for at least three months. Reevaluate to see whether you can reduce sodium even more. Follow your reduced-sodium approach for at least another three months. Repeat the sequence until you have attained your personal nadir of salt consumption.

Visit __www.CardioSmart.org__ for more tips for healthier eating

If you do all the things outlined above, you will likely attain a significant improvement in your blood pressure readings, regardless of your starting point.

Delightful de-pressuring

You can expect these improvements in systolic blood pressure readings associated with recommended lifestyle modifications —

Losing weight	5–20 mmHg decrease per 20 lbs weight lost
Eating a healthy diet	8–14 mmHg decrease
Reducing sodium	2–8 mmHg decrease
Regular physical activity	4–9 mmHg decrease
Reducing alcohol consumption	2–4 mmHg decrease

You can realize anywhere from a 20 to 55 mmHg drop by simply changing your life. That's the same results you'd get from being on a bunch of medications! Doing your part is essential in the battle against this lurking silent killer.

But part of this entire process also involves monitoring where you are and where you're getting to with all your efforts (without or with medications).

Do it yourself

Blood pressure monitoring is something you should undertake in collaboration with your physician. In adults, blood pressure checks should be performed at least yearly. More frequent measurements are required if readings are elevated or significant health changes occur.

You can become more active in measuring and monitoring your blood pressure by investing in a home BP monitor. This is especially important if you have been noted to have elevated or abnormal readings in your doctor's office. Providing your physician with a record of your blood pressures at various times of the day can help him or her assess your blood pressure profile and your response to any interventions or medications. You don't have to become obsessed with taking your readings a million times a day. Ask your health-care provider how many times you should check your readings and when.

Home blood pressure checks can provide vital information, and might completely alter a patient's care plan. I recently consulted on the case of an elderly patient who was complaining of lightheadedness and near-fainting spells. She had been under treatment for high blood pressure for several months with little improvement in her readings, despite progressive increases in her medications. When I saw the patient in my office, her blood pressure reading was 174/90 mmHg. She was reluctant to increase her medications further. I asked her to obtain a blood pressure monitor for home and keep track of her readings over a couple of weeks, being sure to take at least some of the readings during the time she was feeling lightheaded. I was concerned that perhaps some of her pressure readings were even higher and contributing to her symptoms. And I was hoping that the blood pressure data would help me to convince her that she needed more medications.

When she returned with her blood pressure diary, we were both surprised at her readings. Most of her BP values were well below 130/80 mmHg, and during times of lightheadedness, actually fell below 100 mmHg systolic. We checked her monitor against the blood pressure cuff in the office; both gave the same reading — 174/88 mmHg. It turns out that this particular patient displayed what is referred to as "white-coat hypertension" — blood pressure readings that are elevated simply due to being in a doctor's office, but not necessarily reflective of readings outside of the office. The patient's lightheadedness was not due to markedly elevated readings, but rather readings that were too low for her. Once we discontinued her blood pressure medications, her lightheadedness completely resolved and she remained with readings well below 140/80 mmHg on her home monitor. In the office, her readings remained in the 170/90 mmHg range.

No place like home

The opposite can also be true. Patients who have borderline or mildly elevated readings in the office can turn out to have much higher readings during the rest of the day, indicating the need for commencing or adjusting antihypertensive therapy.

If the blood pressure readings are completely normal in the office, there is usually little need for monitoring blood pressures at home.

There are many options for home BP monitoring including a large selection of automated cuffs. Some of these are very similar to blood pressure cuffs used in your doctor's office. Ask your physician if he or she has any recommendations. Your pharmacist is also a good resource for helping you choose the model that fits your lifestyle and budget. (A typical home monitor ranges in price from $20 to $100, with higher prices for the most automated models.) *Consumer Reports* also rates BP monitoring devices — you could use that as a reference guide. You should start your blood pressure evaluation in your doctor's office; if you need closer follow-up of your BP readings, ask your doctor about home monitoring options.

Whichever unit you choose, a *vital* step is to bring the monitor into your doctor's office to make sure that the readings you get on your home monitor are accurate and consistent with the office readings.

Numerous blood pressure medications are available. If you need medications to control your pressures, your physician will have many options at their disposal for attaining optimal results. But be involved in your care. If you are seeing readings at your checkups that are over 120/80 mmHg, and especially over 130/85 mmHg, discuss these readings with your health-care provider and analyze how you might improve these readings.

When it comes to controlling elevated blood pressures, physicians concentrate on making sure that the systolic reading is in the appropriate range. Normalizing your systolic pressure appears to have the most health benefit. So as you are working with your health-care provider to attain good readings, pay special attention to your "top number."

Piece of Advice #9

Keep a diary of your blood pressure readings. At the very least keep a log of the blood pressures obtained when you have had a physical performed. Talk to your doctor about readings consistently over 130/85 mmHg and especially over 140/90 mmHg. *You can slay this giant!*

Visit www.CardioSmart.org for more tips and information to help you track and lower your blood pressure

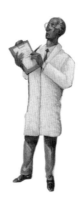

CHAPTER 12

Up in Flames

Smoking is one of the leading causes of statistics.
— FLETCHER KNEBEL

T his chapter is not going to be very long — because there is only one thing to say:

If you smoke, you must quit!

That's it. We're done now. If you like, you can skip ahead to the next chapter.

Tobacco use remains the single most preventable cause of death, especially as it relates to heart disease. Estimates are that smoking directly causes 400,000 deaths in the United States per year.

Kill you, kill me

And if you need another sobering thought:

Anywhere from 35,000 to 65,000 people die of secondhand smoke per year. Secondhand smoke not only increases the risk of developing heart disease and lung cancer, but also increases the risk of young women developing breast cancer and the risk of pregnant women giving birth prematurely. It also increases the rates of asthma.

So if you smoke, you're not only killing yourself, you're killing the people around you. And if you smoke around your children ... you should know better!

Smoking "a little" is not an excuse. I have patients who tell me they are "social smokers," or "party smokers," or "smoke just on the weekends." That's like being a "little" pregnant.

The effects of tobacco smoke are immediate — smoking causes constriction of your arteries (remember how normal arteries can dilate in response to exercise? Tobacco blocks that mechanism), and the components of tobacco smoke are toxic to the endothelium. The products in tobacco also lower HDL levels, increase the number of oxidized and more toxic LDL particles, and make the blood more prone to clotting.

If you combine narrower arteries, vulnerable endothelium, and thicker blood, you can see how tobacco creates the perfect storm for the development of a heart attack. By reducing protective HDL levels and making the LDL more toxic and the endothelium more vulnerable to injury, tobacco use also leads to increased plaque formation and gunk deposition over time.

Smoking puts you at risk for both the chronic buildup of gunk inside your arteries and for the sudden development of a devastating cardiovascular event.

Happily, quitting smoking can result in rapid, dramatic changes in this picture. The artery-narrowing, endothelium-toxic, blood-clotting effects of tobacco are reduced within 24 hours of stopping smoking. However, it takes many years of abstinence to equalize an ex-smoker's risk of developing heart disease with that of people who have never smoked.

The effects of quitting on cancer risk are less rosy. The imparted risk of smoking is cumulative and does not regress even if you stop smoking. If you have smoked, you are at a greater risk for developing cancer than you'd be if you hadn't smoked. The rate of rise in risk declines when you stop smoking, but you can't erase the damage that has already been done. *The sooner you stop smoking the better!*

Being admonished to quit and actually quitting are two different things — and one is infinitely easier than the other. Clearly, simple advice is not always easy to follow.

Be a quitter

Both of my parents were heavy smokers. One day, my father decided to quit — he put down his cigarettes and never smoked again. He was the ultimate cold-turkey quitter. For some of you, quitting can be that simple. For others, quitting is much more difficult.

My mother had a very difficult time stopping smoking. She had witnessed my father deal with cigarettes definitively and instantly, but going cold turkey didn't work for her, despite multiple attempts. And this was long before nicotine gum or patches. What finally clicked was an organized program run in a shopping mall, not far from our home in Toronto. This program worked by helping quitters dissociate smoking from those activities that triggered their cravings.

If you think about it, a good deal of smoking occurs not because someone craves a cigarette in and of itself, but because the act of smoking has become a ritualized component of another behavior. Pick up the phone

— light up. Get in the car — light up. Drink a cup of coffee — light up. The program helped my mother to progressively break these associations. As I remember it, in the first week of the program, my mother was not allowed to smoke while talking on the phone. If she was talking on the phone and craved a cigarette, she had to finish the conversation and hang up. Then she could smoke a pack if she wanted to, but she could no longer smoke during a telephone conversation. The next week, no smoking while driving was added. Again, if she was driving a car and needed to smoke, she would have to pull over to the side of the road and get out of the car to light up. Again, the number of cigarettes she could smoke was not necessarily limited — as long as the smoking did not take place with the targeted activities.

Over time, my mother's opportunities to smoke became more and more restricted, and she smoked less and less. Finally, she was lighting up so infrequently that it was easy to stop entirely. This whole process took several weeks — but in the end, she quit successfully and in over 30 years she's never picked up another cigarette.

Worth trying

I'm not implying that this phase-out approach is the miracle cure for everyone. But if you have tried to quit smoking and have been unsuccessful, maybe an approach like this is worth trying.

Another approach: gradually reducing the number of cigarettes you smoke by one or two cigarettes per day each week. So if you start out smoking a pack a day, get down to 19 or 18 a day for a week or so and then reduce again. Don't trust yourself to not smoke the last couple of cigarettes in the pack — destroy them at the beginning of the day so that they aren't there as a late-day bonus or stashed for "emergency" use. Yes, it's expensive and wasteful to destroy cigarettes (especially if you're down to five a day and you begin each day by crumbling and tossing 15 out of the pack), but you're not spending any more than you would if you were still smoking a pack a day. And destroying the cigarettes is a much better option than having the cigarettes destroy *you*.

How to quit

Many resources are available to help you quit. Among these are —

- Many health insurance companies have programs or can recommend another program close to you.

- The American Lung Association has print and Web-based information about quitting smoking and on smoking cessation programs in your community.

- Your local hospital probably runs a smoking cessation program or has listings of programs in the area.

- Your physician should also be able to direct you to programs in your community and be willing to discuss options for nicotine replacement products and medications to assist in smoking cessation.

- SmokEnders — in your local community or visit www. smokenders.com.

Quitting smoking is one of the best things you can do for yourself, not only to reduce your risk of heart disease but also to reduce your risk of a multitude of cancers. If you do smoke, you absolutely need to muster the willpower and motivation to quit. Every cigarette robs you of a little bit of your life. In fact, here's a sobering thought: *Every cigarette smoked reduces your life expectancy by up to 26 minutes.* And those minutes really count if you're hoping to see your grandchildren graduate from college!

If you were a smoker but have quit — congratulations! You have made a truly positive step toward avoiding disease. If you were in my office, I would be giving you a high-five.

Piece of Advice #10

A multitude of resources are out there to help you quit smoking. Set a quit date, meet with your physician to discuss your plan of action, and use all the resources available to be successful in quitting smoking and staying smoke free. Quit smoking now! You can do this!

Piece of Advice #11

If you've quit smoking in the past, but then started again — don't beat yourself up. The fact that you were able to quit once means that you *can* quit! That's a *huge* positive. It's likely that you will be successful quitting again. The best thing you can do is analyze what prompted you to resume smoking and see how you can avoid that same situation in the future. Quit smoking now! You can do this!

CHAPTER 13

How Sweet It Is!

*Sham Harga had run a successful eatery for many years
by always smiling, never extending credit,
and realizing that most of his customers wanted meals
properly balanced between the four food groups:
sugar, starch, grease, and burnt crunchy bits.*
— Terry Pratchett

Jackie Gleason was an icon. He will always be remembered as Ralph Kramden, the loveable bus driver prone to get-rich-quick schemes and lapses in common sense. He was a big, jolly fellow — and the poster child for adult-onset **diabetes**.

Some diabetics are thin and develop diabetes in childhood. They have a disease in which specific insulin-producing cells reduce production of this hormone. Insulin levels begin to fall, which causes blood sugar levels to rise. Simply put, this type of diabetes, often called **type 1**, is a problem of *insulin supply*. Because our cells need sugar to live, people with this condition require insulin shots to absorb the sugar in their blood. Without insulin, they can't "feed" their cells and they die. There is not much that anyone can do to prevent this type of diabetes. It just happens. We don't understand why. This form of diabetes accounts for 5 to 10 percent of all diabetes in our country. Significant strides have been made in the treatment of this disorder, but currently there is no cure.

Demand in type 2

The vast majority of diabetics (90 to 95 percent) in our country are overweight and develop the disease in adulthood. This is the type of diabetes often associated with Ralph Kramden's appearance — round, especially in the middle. Under these circumstances, people become diabetic not because they stop producing insulin, but because their bodies become progressively less sensitive to the insulin that circulates in their blood. This type of diabetes, often called **type 2**, is a problem of *insulin demand*.

As we eat more and more, we release more and more insulin to help store the sugars and nutrients circulating in our blood vessels. As this goes on for an extended period of time, our cells (which store the sugar) become progressively less responsive to the insulin that is always around. We develop a *tolerance* to the insulin — just as you might develop a tolerance to painkillers or to alcohol — such that we require progressively more and more insulin to achieve the same biochemical effect. Eventually, our ability to produce enough insulin is outpaced by the cells' resistance to the insulin, causing blood sugar to rise.

But just as it takes a long time and a lot of accumulation to go from plaque buildup to chest pain, so it takes a long time to go from high insulin levels to full-blown diabetes. So just because your blood sugars are OK does *not* mean you are necessarily biochemically stellar. Insulin balance can be off (even dramatically so) and may not be discovered by routine testing. If you are overweight but have normal blood sugars, don't pat yourself on the back just yet!

Lips to hips

Why care about elevated insulin levels? You have heard me say over and over again that insulin is a storage hormone. It puts our bodies into storage mode. But it's probably not just blood sugar and cholesterol that are affected — it's a generalized shift in biochemistry. When you have excess insulin bathing your tissues day in and day out (even if your blood sugars are completely normal), you might also become a *calorie hoarder*, and put the calories you take in on a fast track "from the lips to the hips."

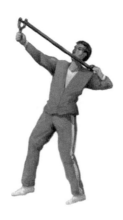

"Pow! Right in the kisser!"

Abnormally elevated blood sugar levels are common, affecting approximately *one in five* Americans. Here's why that's important, as detailed in this chapter —

- Chronically elevated glucose levels lead to blood vessel, nerve, and organ damage. The number one cause of death in diabetics is cardiovascular disease.

- An abnormal fasting glucose level is defined as any number above 100 mg/dL. Repeated values above 125 mg/dL define the presence of full-blown diabetes.

- Even intermediate FBG levels (those between 100 and 125 mg/dL) are very worrisome and require an all-out effort to reverse this abnormality.

- The vast majority of diabetics have type 2 diabetes, which is closely linked to excess weight and lack of physical activity.

- Even in the absence of blood sugar abnormalities, excess weight alters our biochemistry in serious ways, with weight gain promoting more weight gain.

- If your sugars are elevated, work with your physician and your health-care team to bring those values down ASAP.

- If you are overweight (even if your blood sugars are normal) make weight loss an immediate priority. The longer you wait, the harder it will be to lose the weight you need to lose.

- If you don't act now, this disease and all its complications will creep up on you in no time. And before you know it, it'll strike. As Jackie Gleason said, "Pow! Right in the kisser!"

As we get older and our metabolism generally slows down, the excess insulin effect is magnified and it becomes even more difficult to lose weight. This is why it is vital to do everything you can to slim down (if you need to) ASAP. The sooner you start battling your insulin levels the better. And be absolutely vigilant about your children's eating habits and weight status — you don't want to be raising insulin addicts.

I need to clarify something here. When it comes to insulin levels, I am not advocating a low carbohydrate existence. I will talk about dietary choices and food strategies in the chapter about diet. My point is that all excess weight — and especially weight gain around your middle section — causes high insulin levels in general, and places you on track for more weight gain.

Get off the merry-go-round! Balance your calorie intake, move your body, slay that giant! And understand that if you are significantly overweight you'll need greater effort and more persistence (at least initially) because of your altered biochemistry. But don't give up! Your persistence *will* pay off. I promise.

Getting back to diabetes ...

Killing you sweetly

The common issue for type 1 and type 2 diabetics is excess blood sugar floating around in the blood stream. And that excess blood sugar causes health problems over time. Excess blood sugar can ruin small blood vessels, causing the development of small hemorrhages. This is not a big deal if the hemorrhage is in your skin. It IS a big deal if it happens in your eye or in your brain. Excess sugar can also cause nerve endings to degenerate. And that can cause loss of feeling or constant pain. (Obviously, neither is desirable.) Excess sugar also causes kidney disease and kidney failure over time. But the most damaging effect of excess sugar is that it promotes atherosclerosis.

Excess sugar kills — slowly, but relentlessly. And the number one killer of diabetics is cardiovascular disease. It's as if the giant picks out diabetics preferentially to club and throw into the river. To him, they are especially easy prey.

Whether you're a type 1 or type 2 diabetic, the end result is the same. You have abnormally high levels of blood sugar (glucose) circulating in your blood stream. And under both scenarios, you require help to reduce those glucose levels. Type 1 diabetics need insulin shots to accomplish this. (Remember, they're not making much insulin to begin with.) At present, this type of diabetes is permanent and irreversible. Type 2 diabetics can get by with pill-form medications, but over time may also require insulin shots if glucose levels remain difficult to control. For many type 2 diabetics, however, the disease is often reversible and can be completely controlled with lifestyle changes — especially weight loss.

Unfortunately, we are becoming progressively fatter as a nation, and more and more of us are developing type 2 diabetes. This devastation must stop. We have to turn the tide — now — before we're all blind, in pain and on dialysis.

Scary as cancer

Currently there are over 20 *million* diabetics in our country and those numbers are growing. And type 2 diabetes is beginning to affect younger and younger people. In years past, it was rare to see a diabetic child with anything other than the type 1 form of the disease. Now type 2 diabetes is not uncommon in childhood. Why? Because our children are fat, too.

And remember: Even though you have normal blood sugars, you may not necessarily be in the clear if you are also overweight. You could be under the spell of high insulin levels and all the negative, downstream effects of this excess.

What if I told you that you had terminal cancer and that your doctors could offer no cures — just some drugs that might temporarily slow the spread of the disease. What if I then told you that if you lost weight, you could attain complete remission of the cancer, that this would be a cure, a way to keep the cancer at bay and from significantly affecting your life expectancy. Wouldn't you run right out of my office and lose that weight?

Understandably, patients are scared to death of the word "cancer," but I must admit that I find it difficult to comprehend why patients who are overweight and have type 2 diabetes don't immediately lose the weight that's causing their disease. Diabetes can be just as devastating as cancer and can reduce your life expectancy to a similar degree. No doubt losing weight is difficult and requires a real commitment — but we're talking about saving your life here! Isn't an all-out effort paramount?

Some risk factors for developing type 2 diabetes over time cannot be modified. Being Hispanic, Native American, African-American, Asian-American, or Pacific Islander increases the risk. Having a family history of diabetes increases the risk. And diabetes is more likely to develop as we get older. Women who have experienced high blood sugars during pregnancy also face an increased risk of developing diabetes down the road. But the main factors for most of us are excess weight and lack of exercise. If you have any of the non-modifiable risks for developing diabetes, you have to be even more obsessed with your diet and exercise routine. For the rest of us, when it comes to preventing diabetes, a little obsession would also be a good thing.

How sweet it isn't

How do you know if you have diabetes? The best way to find this out is through a blood test that measures your blood sugar levels. This test is performed after you have been fasting for at least 12 hours. A normal **fasting blood glucose (FBG)** level falls below 100 mg/dL. Levels between 100 and 125 mg/dL indicate the presence of pre-diabetes, and levels at 126 mg/dL or above indicate that diabetes is present.

Occasionally, doctors perform what is called the **oral glucose tolerance test**. After fasting, the patient is given a predetermined amount of a sweetened beverage to drink. Two hours later, blood sugar is measured via a blood test. Glucose levels below 140 mg/dL are considered normal.

Levels between 140 and 199 mg/dL are consistent with pre-diabetes, and levels at or above 200 mg/dL indicate that diabetes is present.

I've just thrown in a term into the discussion — "prediabetes." **Prediabetes** is the situation in which a patient's blood sugars are not normal, but they're not high enough to fit the criteria for diabetes per se. Over 40 million people in the United States fit the definition of prediabetes. So over 60 million people — about *one-fifth* of all the people in this country — are walking around with abnormal blood sugars. And countless more are walking around with abnormal insulin levels. Pretty staggering statistics, don't you think?

Even though "prediabetes" sounds less ominous than "diabetes," it is a very serious condition and can be associated with long-term health effects and accelerated rates of heart and vascular disease. Every person who develops type 2 diabetes first goes through prediabetes (and everyone first goes through elevated insulin levels before they become prediabetic). The general estimate is that once you have been diagnosed with prediabetes, developing type 2 diabetes is on average 10 years away. (I have no estimate of the time line between high insulin levels and prediabetes, but suspect it would be in the same range.) But guess what? Through diet and exercise, you can completely prevent the development of prediabetes and type 2 diabetes. Here's the recipe:

> *High-fiber, low-saturated-fat, calorie-balanced food consumption. Daily exercise. Weight loss.*

I know I'm a broken record. And I know you know this stuff already. So what are you waiting for? Get going!

Glucose glut

Here are your immediate steps if you …

- already have type 2 diabetes: Go look at yourself in the mirror. If you are overweight, make a contract with yourself to lose the weight you need to lose, to change what you consume and to increase your exercise. There is no time to waste. Your blood vessels, your nerve endings and your organs are all suffering in the sugar bath. Take back your life!

- have prediabetes: *There is no time to waste.* You must make every effort to reverse the trend that's taking you down the path to medications and insulin injections.

- are overweight: Lose the weight you need to lose. Increase your exercise levels. Change your diet. Act now to change your destiny.

- don't know what your blood sugar is: For heaven's sake — get tested! Having a fasting blood glucose level should be part of your general physical evaluation.

Piece of Advice #12

Having your fasting blood glucose level evaluated at every general physical, and yearly exam after the age of 50, is a must. If any of your readings fall into the pre-diabetes range, you will need to have your glucose levels tested more frequently than that. Talk to your doctor about a reasonable monitoring schedule *for you*. If you are diabetic, and especially if you need insulin, you will need to test your glucose levels at least daily, and probably several times per day. Regardless of your testing schedule, keep track of your readings. This is your body. You are in the best position to serve as the keeper of your "maintenance" information.

Elevated blood sugars can occur *without any symptoms* — especially in the pre-diabetes stage. So you could be walking around with elevated glucose levels without knowing it. Once you become diabetic, you may experience increased thirst, more frequent urination, fatigue and/or blurred vision if the condition goes untreated. But even with full-blown diabetes, you might not experience symptoms to give you a clue that you have the disease. This is why it's important to have periodic blood sugar checks.

Whether you have diabetes or prediabetes, keeping your blood sugar as close to normal as possible can significantly affect the occurrence of complications from this disease.

Go figure sugar

One way to measure your overall blood sugar control is with a test called **glycosylated hemoglobin (HbA1c**, pronounced "hemoglobin-A-one-C"). Hemoglobin is found within our red blood cells and is involved in oxygen transport. Glucose attaches itself to hemoglobin in proportion to blood sugar levels, resulting in hemoglobin that is "glycosylated." Unlike regular blood glucose levels (which measure blood sugar control in the immediate present), the measurement of glycosylated hemoglobin reflects overall blood sugar control over a longer period — over the past couple of months. It's like an average of all the blood sugars you have had every minute of the day over the past 60 to 90 days.

Knowing this number can be very useful. Because individual blood sugar measurements depend on so many different factors — food composition, activity level, intrinsic insulin production, extrinsic medication, or insulin administration — a single blood sugar measurement (or even several) may not provide an accurate picture of overall blood sugar control.

The HbA1C, by providing us with an assessment of average control, gives us a much better understanding of your overall blood sugar burden. Normal HbA1C levels fall below 6 percent. Patients with diabetes should strive to keep their HbA1C levels below 7 percent. If your HbA1C levels fall above 7 percent, your blood sugar levels are excessively high too much of the time.

Diabetes control and blood sugar management are not undertakings you should attempt on your own. If you have diabetes or pre-diabetes, work closely with your doctor and health-care team to normalize your glucose readings and to minimize any factors that may be contributing to your **hyperglycemia** (high sugar readings). But just as with high blood pressure, don't accept the plan to merely watch your readings. Ask for advice about your condition — and then follow that advice. Do your part by becoming more physically active, reducing calorie intake (if your are overweight), and being more mindful of the types of foods you eat.

Dieticians, nutritionists, diabetes specialists — these individuals are all available and skilled at helping you control your diabetes or elevated blood sugar levels. Get active and get involved. Keep track of your blood sugar readings and watch for progressive increases in those readings — especially if you fall into the prediabetes category.

But remember: When it comes to type 2 diabetes and prediabetes, those dieticians, nutritionists, diabetes specialists and your personal physician can only help delay the effects of this disease. Only *you* have the power to get it into remission.

If you are overweight and reading this chapter — and your blood sugars are normal — don't take those numbers as a sign that your body is tolerating your excess weight. You are setting yourself up for more and more weight gain and the eventual appearance of high blood sugars. Alter your destiny. *Now.*

CHAPTER 14

"Mommy, that lady is really fat!"

Now there are more overweight people in
America than average-weight people.
So overweight people are now average.
Which means you've met your
New Year's resolution.

— Jay Leno

Imagine my horror when my four-year-old son yelled this out (at what seemed to be the top of his lungs) about three feet away from a woman in a grocery store. If the floor of the store could have opened up — where I was standing, at that very moment — I would have been grateful. Instead I was left to turn positively beet red with embarrassment and to apologize as best I could to the poor woman, who happened to be in the wrong place at the wrong time.

Fat nation

In all fairness to my child, the woman *was* fat. And he was only observing as unusual what most of us have come to accept as ordinary. The truth? America is turning into a fat nation!

This is not just a matter of how we look — this is also a matter of how long we live. Studies have shown that the risk of death increases with increasing weight. Even moderate excess weight (10 to 20 pounds) increases the risk of early death. How much risk? Well, it's estimated that in America 300,000 deaths a year may be attributable to obesity.

If you're a young adult (in your 20s or early 30s), are five feet four inches tall and weigh over 260 pounds, or six feet tall and weigh over 330 pounds, your life span is expected to be reduced by at least 20 *years* due to your weight alone. Yes, those weight/height combinations are extreme — but they're becoming more and more common. In this land of plenty, we are literally eating ourselves into our graves.

Here are a couple of maps that may help open your eyes to what is happening to the population in our country.

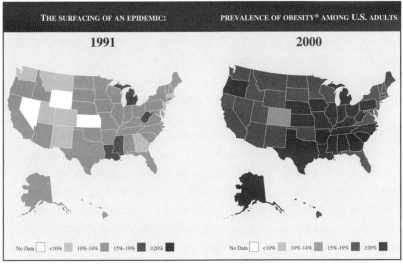

Source: Surgeon General's Call to Action to Prevent and Decrease Overweight and Obesity, published in 2001.

When I saw these maps for the first time, my heart sank. This wasn't a minor change in the weight and appearance of Americans. *This was a dramatic shift over a very short period of time.* And I bet the statistics are even worse today. Something bad is happening with respect to how we live our lives, how we eat and how we treat our bodies! How did we get here? And how do we get back?

The why of obesity

Obesity and being overweight are caused by many factors. Every overweight person brings different factors to the table — genetic differences, metabolic differences, cultural differences, behavioral and environmental differences. The latter two — behavioral and environmental factors — are responsible for an especially large part of the problem.

I look at our children and worry. Adults have adopted bad habits and are transmitting them to their offspring, setting the stage for an even more overweight generation to come. We have stopped modeling good-food behaviors, and it's really showing. If we eat on the run, eat convenience foods, decrease our fresh fruit and vegetable intake, and eat out more and more, we can't possibly expect our children to behave any differently.

When I talk to my patients and my friends, I find similar themes emerging over and over. We are spending more and more time running around, shuttling ourselves and our children to an increasingly overwhelming number of activities and trying to balance all these duties with increasing work demands. Stay-at-home moms are largely women of the past (even if some moms are not part of the traditional workforce, they're still never home), and traveling for work is more common than ever. Something's got to give — and it's set mealtimes and home cooking. When you eat irregularly and on the go, it gets very difficult to track your intake, both in terms of calories and in terms of nutritional value.

The price of low cost

Another theme is the rising cost of food. I am forever struck by how much more I seem to spend to buy less. And if I buy expensive organic produce and seafood that ends up spoiling in my refrigerator because my family won't eat it or I don't have time to prepare it, well ... it'll be a while before I spend my money that way again. So the variety of products I purchase narrows and tends toward foods that won't spoil and that I know my kids will eat. That's convenience food, extra sugary or salty food, and ready or partially prepared food — food especially high in calories and low in nutritional value. It's the food that dominates most grocery shelves and fast food chains — and that tends to be less expensive.

And when I use "my family" and "I" in the paragraph above, I *really* mean my family and me. I may be a cardiologist and "know better," but I can still be human — and my children can still like junk food and refuse to try anything new. Maybe you can relate if this happens to you. But just because we can relate, and just because my family falls into this food trap at times, doesn't mean that it is acceptable or should be excused in any way.

By the way, when I see myself falling into this pattern, I step back and really make an effort to return to the good food habits I know I should follow and model for my children. Often that involves not only changing what I buy at the store, but also changing aspects of my life around a bit so that I can be home more often to prepare food and be there with my family to eat the meals. And sometimes it takes cutting down on activities so that my children can be home as well.

Weighty facts

- Obesity and excess weight are extremely common in our society and associated with a multitude of health risks and a shortened life span.

- To assess your own status, use the Body Mass Index table to determine your body mass index. Anything over 25 is concerning. Anything over 30 is a *weight emergency*.

- Your waist measurement is another clue to impending disaster. Forty inches or more in a man and 35 inches or more in a woman are calls for immediate action.

- There are no magic solutions to get rid of excess weight — it's calories in versus calories out. If you take in more than you expend, you will gain weight. The only way to lose weight is to eat less and move more.

We must look inward

Portion size has gotten out of control and we have lost perspective about what constitutes a normal serving. By eating out more and allowing others to decide how much should land on our plates, we set ourselves up for calorie overload. And we progressively alter our expectations of what constitutes a real meal "value." What is valuable is the *quality* of the food not the *quantity* of the food. Getting a lot doesn't mean that it's smart to eat what you get.

We exercise less. We commute by car, spend our time sitting in front of computers at work, and come home to watch TV. We don't walk anywhere because the suburbs in which we live don't have sidewalks, and anything we'd want to walk to is miles away. We worry for our children if they go riding their bikes outside, but we're too tired to go biking with them. We buy them video games and put them on buses to school. And we take away physical education classes so that our towns can balance their school budgets.

So forces are out there — multiple forces — that conspire against us and against our efforts to live healthy and calorie-balanced lives. But we must look inward as well as outward — because a lot of these forces are self-inflicted and self-perpetuated. And the truth is undeniable — we are getting fatter and fatter and fatter.

How to know if you are overweight or obese? By seeing where you fit on the BMI table. **BMI** stands for "body mass index" and it is a measure that relates weight to height. The actual formula is this:

> BMI = [Weight in Pounds / (Height in inches) x (Height in inches)] x 703

Body Mass Index Table

BMI	19	20	21	22	23	24	25	26	27	28	29	30	31	32	33	34	35	36
Height (inches)	**Body Weight (pounds)**																	
58	91	96	100	105	110	115	119	124	129	134	138	143	148	153	158	162	167	172
59	94	99	104	109	114	119	124	128	133	138	143	148	153	158	163	168	173	178
60	97	102	107	112	118	123	128	133	138	143	148	153	158	163	168	174	179	184
61	100	106	111	116	122	127	132	137	143	148	153	158	164	169	174	180	185	190
62	104	109	115	120	126	131	136	142	147	153	158	164	169	175	180	186	191	196
63	107	113	118	124	130	135	141	146	152	158	163	169	175	180	186	191	197	203
64	110	116	122	128	134	140	145	151	157	163	169	174	180	186	192	197	204	209
65	114	120	126	132	138	144	150	156	162	168	174	180	186	192	198	204	210	216
66	118	124	130	136	142	148	155	161	167	173	179	186	192	198	204	210	216	223
67	121	127	134	140	146	153	159	166	172	178	185	191	198	204	211	217	223	230
68	125	131	138	144	151	158	164	171	177	184	190	197	203	210	216	223	230	236
69	128	135	142	149	155	162	169	176	182	189	196	203	209	216	223	230	236	243
70	132	139	146	153	160	167	174	181	188	195	202	209	216	222	229	236	243	250
71	136	143	150	157	165	172	179	186	193	200	208	215	222	229	236	243	250	257
72	140	147	154	162	169	177	184	191	199	206	213	221	228	235	242	250	258	265
73	144	151	159	166	174	182	189	197	204	212	219	227	235	242	250	257	265	272
74	148	155	163	171	179	186	194	202	210	218	225	233	241	249	256	264	272	280
75	152	160	168	176	184	192	200	208	216	224	232	240	248	256	264	272	279	287
76	156	164	172	180	189	197	205	213	221	230	238	246	254	263	271	279	287	295

BMI	37	38	39	40	41	42	43	44	45	46	47	48	49	50	51	52	53	54
Height (inches)	**Body Weight (pounds)**																	
58	177	181	186	191	196	201	205	210	215	220	224	229	234	239	244	248	253	258
59	183	188	193	198	203	208	212	217	222	227	232	237	242	247	252	257	262	267
60	189	194	199	204	209	215	220	225	230	235	240	245	250	255	261	266	271	276
61	195	201	206	211	217	222	227	232	238	243	248	254	259	264	269	275	280	285
62	202	207	213	218	224	229	235	240	246	251	256	262	267	273	278	284	289	295
63	208	214	220	225	231	237	242	248	254	259	265	270	278	282	287	293	299	304
64	215	221	227	232	238	244	250	256	262	267	273	279	285	291	296	302	308	314
65	222	228	234	240	246	252	258	264	270	276	282	288	294	300	306	312	318	324
66	229	235	241	247	253	260	266	272	278	284	291	297	303	309	315	322	328	334
67	236	242	249	255	261	268	274	280	287	293	299	306	312	319	325	331	338	344
68	243	249	256	262	269	276	282	289	295	302	308	315	322	328	335	341	348	354
69	250	257	263	270	277	284	291	297	304	311	318	324	331	338	345	351	358	365
70	257	264	271	278	285	292	299	306	313	320	327	334	341	348	355	362	369	376
71	265	272	279	286	293	301	308	315	322	329	338	343	351	358	365	372	379	386
72	272	279	287	294	302	309	316	324	331	338	346	353	361	368	375	383	390	397
73	280	288	295	302	310	318	325	333	340	348	355	363	371	378	386	393	401	408
74	287	295	303	311	319	326	334	342	350	358	365	373	381	389	396	404	412	420
75	295	303	311	319	327	335	343	351	359	367	375	383	391	399	407	415	423	431
76	304	312	320	328	336	344	353	361	369	377	385	394	402	410	418	426	435	443

Source: National Heart, Lung, and Blood Institute; available online at
http://www.nhlbi.nih.gov/guidelines/obesity/bmi_tbl.htm

A normal BMI is defined as a BMI below 25. The definition of "overweight" is a BMI of 25–29, and "obesity" is defined as any BMI equal to or greater than 30.

Find your height along the left side of the table and your weight in the row corresponding to your height. The column where your weight and height intersect is your BMI column, and tells you your BMI. If you are in one of the columns below 25 — congratulations! If you're above 25, you are with the majority — the vast majority — of people in this country. And you are at increased risk for heart disease, diabetes, hypertension, gallbladder disease, sleep apnea, and arthritis, as well as cancers of the breast, colon, kidney, gallbladder, and endometrium.

Another measure of worrisome excess weight is the waist circumference. A waist circumference over 40 inches for men or over 35 inches for women is a red flag that there are major concerns in the weight department. These values have been shown to identify individuals at very high risk for developing health issues related to obesity. These people would almost certainly have high insulin levels, and would be set up to develop pre-diabetes and full-blown diabetes over time.

OK, how did you get here and how do you get back? It's harsh and inescapable — it's calories in versus calories out. If you are overweight, you got here by either eating poorly or not exercising enough (or most likely both).

And guess what? The solution, the way to get back, is equally as inescapable and equally as harsh — to lose weight you have to eat differently and move more.

So let's take the next two chapters to talk about what you should be eating and how you should be moving. Ready?

CHAPTER 15

"Diet" Is a Four-Letter Word

I've been on a diet for two weeks and all I've lost is two weeks.
— TOTIE FIELDS

How many diets have you been on? Have you been successful at losing weight? How did you feel on those diets? How fun were you to be around?

Here's why diets fail: Ultimately, dieters feel deprived and with deprivation comes want and obsession. We are all too obsessed about food. Somewhere along the line, food went from being a necessity and a pleasure to being an enemy and a punishment. We are either guilt ridden if we enjoy eating something "bad," or try to punish ourselves through deprivation. The balance is gone.

Normal eating

I think we all need to stop dieting and start eating normally. We just have to relearn what *normal* means. Normal is variety. Normal is tasty.

Normal is freshly prepared. Normal is chemical free. Normal is reasonably portioned. Normal is simple. Normal is satisfying. Normal is healthy. Normal is what we already know we should be eating. If there's a pile of potato chips and some cut-up fruit sitting on a counter and you're asked to pick the healthier item, you will almost certainly pick the fruit. We actually know *what* we need to eat — we just don't.

That's the amazing thing. Diet book after diet book hits the bestseller list. And we all go to them looking for the magic bullet — the home run — something fast and easy. Unfortunately, fast and easy are not realistic expectations for good nutrition and sustained weight loss. Pursuing good nutrition is a commitment that's renewed every day, for every meal, for every ingredient. And the formula for weight loss is not magic — a calorie is a calorie is a calorie. And the only way to lose weight is to eat less and move more.

I do have to acknowledge that I will place some of my patients on specific eating plans because I want these people to make dramatic changes and recognize how they can alter their eating patterns within a strict framework — and because I think they will have more success (at least initially) with a regimented plan. But I also try to point them toward a more balanced, long-term approach to food consumption, because for the long haul, you need good food habits, not cookie-cutter diets.

So I'm not going to give you step-by-step eating plans with detailed menus and lists of restrictive food behaviors. I'm going to give you a framework to help you make better choices and be healthier. I'm going to give you *my* recipe for good food habits.

Recipe for Good Food Habits

Here's a quick list of the ingredients in this recipe. Below, you'll find details on every ingredient.

- Ingredient #1: Control portions

- Ingredient #2: Put the fork down when you are full

- Ingredient #3: Don't eat if you're not hungry

- Ingredient #4: Choose quality over quantity

- Ingredient #5: Avoid the extras

- Ingredient #6: Eat in reverse order

- Ingredient #7: Don't snack

- Ingredient #8: Choose smart carb, not low carb

- Ingredient #9: Eat your fruits and vegetables!

- Ingredient #10: Choose smart fat, not low fat

- Ingredient #11: Allow an egg a day (don't obsess over the cholesterol)

- Ingredient #12: Put down the salt shaker

- Ingredient #13: Make food special

- Ingredient #14: Prepare your own food

- Ingredient #15: Never ever eat fast food

- Ingredient #16: Choose your fluids wisely

- Ingredient #17: A calorie is *not* a calorie is *not* a calorie

Ingredient #1: Control portions

Never eat more than you can lift.
— Miss Piggy

The first thing to do — even if you do nothing else (but I hope you make lots of changes beyond this one) — is to become a portion-control hawk. *We eat way too much food!* Many of the single portions that restaurants serve could feed a small family — sometimes even a large one! Be realistic about how much food you really need when ordering and either skip the appetizer or consider getting an appetizer for both the first and main portions of your meals. Sometimes an appetizer is a meal in itself. Use your brain, not your eyes, when ordering food. If in doubt, order one course at a time. Share your dessert. Eventually, restaurants will realize that we don't want or need such huge portions, and they will make them smaller. The value is not in the quantity of food, it's in the quality and the experience of the food.

We really need to retrain ourselves about what constitutes a normal serving size. Lots of strategies can help you with this, one of which is shown in the accompanying box. If you're eating out, stay within these estimates and don't sabotage yourself.

The size of it

Useful aids to determine appropriate portion size include visualizing the following —

- A deck of cards as the size of a serving of meat or fish
- A tennis ball as the size of a serving of fruit
- A fist as the size of a serving of rice or pasta
- A giant dump truck as the size of a serving of vegetables

OK — the last one's a bit silly, but I'm trying to make a point.

If a serving is out of step with normal portions, or you're at a restaurant that typically provides large servings, try dividing your food in half right away; then commit to taking the other half home for a meal on a subsequent day (not as a late night snack!). Or ask for a half portion. Or ask to have the portion split between you and a dining companion. If you're at home, you might want to put only half of what you'd normally put on your plate and start there. Think long and hard before refilling the plate. Commit to always leaving something behind. (No — not just the parsley!) Use a smaller plate for serving your food. Just as our portions are getting out of control, the plates that we use to serve the meals are becoming platters. Make it hard for yourself to pile on the food.

As an initial "gut check" (again, pardon the pun), you can use the sense that you're not getting "good value" from your serving as an indication that it's probably the right amount of food. If the bagel looks too small or the cup of coffee doesn't come with mocha syrup and whipped cream, you're probably on the right track. A half sandwich and a cup of soup *is* enough — especially if the sandwich starts as a 12-inch sub or the soup comes in a "bottomless" bowl.

Ingredient #2: Put the fork down when you are full

Learn to listen to your body. If you feel like you are fatigued after a meal, chances are good that you have eaten too much. Aim to eliminate that stuffed feeling completely from your existence.

Eat more slowly — give your body time to figure out if it's had enough. When your body tells you it's full, respect that. Stop eating at that point, even if your eyes want more. A good strategy to follow is to put your fork down several times during the meal. Take a couple of breaths and wait a bit. You may find that this short respite allows you time to better assess whether or not you are full.

Ingredient #3: Don't eat if you're not hungry

Thou shouldst eat to live; not live to eat.
— Socrates (469 BC–399 BC)

Many of us eat not because we're hungry but because it's "something to do" or it's "comforting." Eating should be motivated by the need for nutritional sustenance, rather than by emotion or boredom. All of us are emotional eaters to some extent. Recognizing when you fall into this pattern is a huge step toward changing your behavior. Sometimes, the pattern is followed so subconsciously that you need to keep a food diary to see it. So if you are having difficulty losing the weight you need to lose, keep a food diary to see if you have any eating behaviors and food triggers that may be derailing your efforts.

If you are faced with a lot of business meals, consider your health as well as your obligation to be a good host or congenial guest. Eating massive amounts of food will no more guarantee closing the deal than will wearing a particular pair of socks. Search out the lighter and smaller options on the menu and order according to your appetite and hunger status. Your hosts or guests will understand your attempts to be more healthy. You might even start a trend!

Ingredient #4: Choose quality over quantity

I have come to recognize that (especially when it comes to takeout food), in general, *the less expensive it is, the less of it you should have.* Just because the meal is a good deal for your pocketbook doesn't mean it's a good choice for your health. Really examine what's hitting your mouth.

There's a reason why a small piece of grass-fed organic steak is so much more expensive than a fast-food hamburger. The organic grass-fed sirloin is more expensive to bring to market because the cattle are raised in smaller numbers and with more direct human involvement in their care, and because the cows have to have room to roam and crops need to be rotated to maintain the integrity of their pasture (and all of this costs money).

Think how different the conditions have to be to get beef at pennies per pound for a hamburger chain. The feed, the conditions under which the cows are raised, and the parts of the cow used to make the ground beef all have to favor the lowest and cheapest components to arrive at a profitable hamburger (one that has to be packaged, marketed, sold, and served) for under $1. The quality of the beef in those hamburgers can't possibly equal the nutritional and life-sustenance quality of the organic steak.

This is not to imply that eating well has to be expensive. Fresh produce is generally one of the least expensive items in a supermarket (which may be why more and more produce departments are located way in the back of the store — accessed only after you walk past all the prepared foods and snacks). And salads tend to be among the lowest-priced items on restaurant menus.

The reverse is also true: You shouldn't automatically order a giant piece of steak just because it costs a bundle. Eating healthfully does not have to break the bank — it just simply has to be *mindful*.

Ingredient #5: Avoid the extras

Don't automatically accept the breadbasket. You probably didn't come to the restaurant to eat bread. Chances are you don't start your meals at home with a breadbasket, so why should you change that behavior when you are eating out? And just because you *can* have a giant muffin and hash browns with your omelet doesn't mean you *should!*

Ingredient #6: Eat in reverse order

> *Eat breakfast like a king, lunch like a prince,*
> *and dinner like a pauper.*
> — ADELLE DAVIS

Most people consume more calories as the day goes on. I see a lot of patients who skip breakfast, have a relatively light lunch and go crazy at dinner — often ending the day with late-night snacking. *This is the absolute opposite of what you should be doing.* You are much better off having a substantial breakfast, your main meal at lunchtime and a very light dinner.

Breakfast is a must. Breakfast actually stimulates your metabolism so you are more "wasteful" with your calories throughout the rest of the day. If you skip breakfast, your body will be more likely to go into "conservation" mode, holding on to more calories in fear of another "fast." We are essentially created as extremely efficient, adaptable machines. You want to make sure you are leveraging this adaptability to your advantage. So always start your day with a nutritious meal. My standard practice is to have a cup of yogurt with two to three tablespoons of high-fiber cereal, and at least one half cup of fruit. I also have a cup or two of black or green tea. I feel great and my body is ready to go!

If you face a lot of business meals as part of your daily life, see whether you can schedule more of those meals as lunches rather than as dinners. You will drink less, eat less, and, after a larger meal in the middle of the day, be less likely to need a large meal at night.

Luncheon portions tend to be smaller. Because you have the rest of the day to deal with, you are much less likely to order a multitude of courses and more likely to skip dessert. Whereas we tend to approach dinner out as a major treat and a time to indulge, we tend to see lunch more as a respite from a busy day and not necessarily as an invitation to go over the top in terms of our food consumption.

If anything, you should feel a bit hungry as you go to bed. If you go to bed feeling stuffed or exhausted from the meal you just ate, you have the wrong eating pattern.

Give yourself a break(fast)

This is a long chapter chock full of great advice for long-term healthy eating. However, depending on where you're starting from, it can seem overwhelming to make the changes outlined all at once. There's just so much to remember!

Start by tackling your nutrition one step at a time — one meal at a time.

- *Start with breakfast.* Commit to always having a healthful start to your day. Consider high-fiber cereal with low-fat milk or yogurt, or a couple of boiled eggs with slices of tomato, or high-fiber bread with unsweetened, natural, or organic almond butter or peanut butter.

- *Breakfast is a great time* to include a piece of fruit or a glass of vegetable juice. And remember to have a cup of green tea. Regardless of your location or schedule, commit to always making healthful choices first thing in the morning.

- *For the rest of the day*, at least initially, give yourself a break. Focus on the breakfast. Keep your breakfast commitment for at least two weeks and, when your breakfast routine has truly become routine, add another positive nutrition step, like stopping snacking or tackling your lunches.

- *Read this chapter several times* to make sure that all the concepts sink in and for reinforcement — especially when you see yourself slipping.

- *Be realistic* about goals and expectations. Don't beat yourself up for every indiscretion. But don't give up the whole war when you lose one battle. Just because you eat a couple of cookies doesn't mean you should then eat every sweet or nutritionally vapid food in sight since you've "already blown the day."

Ingredient #7: Don't snack

I'm not sure when snacking became so acceptable. When I was growing up (walking through all that snow, uphill both ways, for miles and miles) we had meals, not snacks. And we didn't eat between meals. Snacks were reserved for parties or days when dinner was significantly delayed for some reason. I never once had a snack at school.

Now it seems we are eating all the time. And it might be OK if we were merely **grazing** (having small amounts of food throughout the day without major meals) — *but that's not what most of us do*. Most of us eat full meals and then munch between those meals, seemingly oblivious to the boatload of calories we are consuming. People who "graze" throughout the day actually tend to be thinner than those who don't. But remember, these individuals are not consuming more calories (even though they may seem to be eating all the time); they are simply spreading out a normal calorie intake throughout the day. Just like people who skip meals train their bodies to be calorie hoarders, people who eat small amounts of food frequently train their bodies to be calorie wasters (because their bodies know that more food is just around the corner).

Getting back to us non-grazers ... Snacking is dangerous because it's almost always mindless. We don't really count it as part of our caloric consumption — a few chips here or a handful of candy there seems too insignificant to worry about. But guess what? Snack foods tend to be calorie-dense foods. So even small amounts add up quickly in terms of calories and (eventually) pounds. Something to keep in mind: **an extra 100 calories per day, translates to a 10-pound weight gain over the course of a year.**

Unless you tend to eat only small meals, are an athlete on a rigorous training schedule, or in the middle of a growth spurt (only vertical growth qualifies!), *stop your snacking ways*. You don't need those calories.

If you *must* eat something between your regular meals, commit to only consuming raw fruits or vegetables. If you absolutely have to have something more substantial, a few nuts should suffice.

Ingredient #8: Choose smart carb, not low carb

Don't deprive yourself of carbohydrates. As a whole, we probably eat way too many simple carbs, but trying to completely eliminate all carbohydrates from our diets is silly. It makes no sense to me that bread, which has been a dietary staple in our societies for several millennia, could ever be labeled as evil!

What matters is not eliminating all carbohydrates, but reducing the bad carbohydrates. What are bad carbohydrates? These are the low-fiber carbohydrates.

I'm not specifically talking about glycemic index here. I am a firm believer that no single food characteristic influences weight gain. I don't believe that carrots could ever be bad for you, even if they are "sweet." For weight gain, it's calories in versus calories out — period.

I am, however, talking about all sugars, white flour, white rice, white pasta, corn syrup, fructose ... You get the idea — carbs that have been extensively processed or refined (stripping them of fiber and micronutrients). These types of carbs do a poor job of suppressing hunger for any great period, and tend to be calorie dense relative to their overall nutritional value. These are the foods and ingredients we should actively limit in our diets.

It's not possible (or necessary) to eliminate them completely. But these are the items we should be on the look out for and ingredients we should try to reduce or substitute with higher-fiber alternatives. So when you eat rice, choose brown or wild rice. When you eat pasta, choose whole-wheat noodles. If you don't like brown rice or whole-wheat pasta, make sure to reduce the portions of white rice and regular pasta you eat (visualize that fist!), and make sure that the accompanying foods (or sauces) are high in fiber (and low in saturated fat).

Pasta and rice

I know what you're thinking: Everyone says the Mediterranean diet is so healthful and they eat a bunch of pasta over there! And then look at the Japanese — they eat white rice all the time and they're not fat! Yes, both of these statements are true. But look closer at the Mediterranean diet. Pasta in Mediterranean countries is served as an appetizer — not as a main course. It comes as a small portion. The main course might be a simple piece of fresh grilled fish served with a few herbs, some olive oil and a sprinkling of lemon juice. No potatoes, no bread. The pasta is essentially a side dish, and doesn't come in a gallon-sized bowl topped with Alfredo sauce. If you love pasta, great! Eat it, enjoy it, but be mindful of the portions and make sure that you get plenty of fiber from other sources. And choose non–cream-based sauces most of the time. And go easy on the cheese.

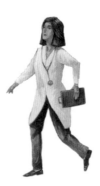

The same goes for the white rice. The Japanese may consume it in conspicuous quantities, but it is essentially the *only* simple carbohydrate they consume and it's balanced by high fiber in the accompanying vegetables, and by the lean protein sources that are all healthfully prepared. It's all a matter of balance.

Bread

What about bread? *It is not evil.* It's not something that you should stop eating. But just as with rice and noodles, make better choices, and reduce your portions. The bread you eat should the densest, heaviest, most sawdust-like bread you can still enjoy — in other words the bread that is highest in fiber. (By the way, just because a bread looks dark doesn't mean it's fiber-full — check the label, ask the breadsmith: You're looking for at least 2 grams of fiber per 100 calories.) And when you have a choice, favor an open-faced sandwich and load up with high-fiber and high-nutrient ingredients like veggies, sprouts and tomatoes.

Maybe you have a bread machine at home that you used to love but that's now collecting dust since you've eliminated bread from your diet. Resurrect that appliance! Find recipes that call for oat bran, wheat germ, flax meal ... Get creative and feed the part of you that craves bread. It's OK, as long as it's fiber-full and you consume it in reasonable quantities (listen to your body!) and at reasonable times (hold that breadbasket!). Eaten this way, bread is perfectly healthy.

Cereal

What about cereal? It's a great food source, and because it is often supplemented with vitamins and minerals and is so easy to prepare it's a perfect choice for folks on the run in the mornings. But some cereals are junk while others are wise choices. Look for high-fiber cereals and for ones low in sugar and other sweeteners. A high-fiber cereal that is heavily sweetened will derail your efforts — you don't need those sugar calories! Food companies have learned that sugar sells, so finding a low-sugar or low-sweetener choice may be difficult. But guess what? If we all start buying lower-sugar cereals, those same companies will give us more choices. If you find a low-sugar but lower-fiber cereal that you like, you can boost the fiber content by sprinkling wheat germ, bran, and/or flax meal over it. Use only skim or low fat milk with your cereal. And eat a reasonable portion.

Cakes, cookies, chocolates, candies —

All bad, right? Not necessarily. **Dark chocolate** (semisweet, bittersweet — look for high cocoa content) is full of flavonoids and other antioxidants and can actually be heart healthy. But in *small* quantities. In my mind, besides fruit, the perfect dessert is a fabulous, solitary piece of dark chocolate, slowly savored. Milk chocolate? You're out of luck. Actually, even having a glass of milk with your dark chocolate appears to nullify the antioxidant effect, so stay away from the milk and chocolate combo.

How about the rest? OK, they are bad — but cakes, cookies, and candies can also taste great and most of us really enjoy eating them. Balance, balance, balance. This is where you have to use some brains and a lot of restraint.

If you're going to consume any one of these items, make sure you:

- Choose something of very high quality and something you truly enjoy — don't eat sweets just because they're around, and don't eat super-processed or preservative-packed junk. It's not just the sugar and calories in those items that are bad for you.

- Use restraint in portion size and don't go for seconds.

- Don't make it a daily habit.

- Balance your intake with better choices in your other foods.

And for goodness sake, stop feeling guilty! Falling into the perpetual guilt and punishment cycle is easy and will only magnify your cravings. If you follow the four steps above, you'll be fine. Allow food to become your friend again.

I have lots of personal experience with this because my mother owns a bakery in Toronto. She makes fabulous pastries, great bread and traditional European doughnuts. Every time I visit I eat anything she serves me, and I always ask for a care package to take home with me. I know how these products are made, I know they are of the highest quality, and I know they taste great! I can't imagine *not* eating them. So I do — but I follow the rules above. You too can be successful at this. If I can do it, anyone can!

Reduced-carbohydrate foods

What about "reduced-carbohydrate" foods? In my mind these are manipulated foods and you may have already gleaned that I'm more in favor of less-processed, less-adulterated choices. The "low-carbohydrate" aspect of these foods usually has to do with the sort of sweetener used. So we're just perpetuating a fraud on our taste buds — and I don't think this is the right solution. We all just simply have to readjust our sweet-meters. Then we won't need the low-carb food options, because less-sweet foods will taste just fine.

If you've ever spent any time in Europe and really delved into local cuisines there, I'm sure you noticed (at least initially) how much sweeter everything tastes upon returning to the United States. Even cakes and pastries are much sweeter in the US than they are in Europe. Chocolate bars are sweeter, salad dressings are sweeter, cereal is sweeter, yogurt is sweeter ... we seem to sweeten everything to the max! After a while, you get used to the taste and it seems normal, but that doesn't mean it is. When shopping, look for items that don't list sugar, sucrose, fructose, glucose, honey, corn syrup, or brown sugar as one of the first two or three ingredients. "Evaporated cane juice" is another phrase for "sugar." Don't fall for labeling tactics — become a thorough reader of ingredient lists. Even items that are touted "low in sugar" may not be "low in sweetness," because they have been artificially enhanced with aspartame or Splenda. Avoid those products, too. Artificial sweetening is *not* the solution for our bulging tummies. The solution is to break our addictions to all things sweet.

Fiber

Getting back to fiber ... Eating a high-fiber diet has multiple benefits — from promoting lower cholesterol levels, to lower insulin levels, to increased satiety, to the elimination of constipation. Fiber causes the slowing of food absorption, leading to fewer and less pronounced blood sugar peaks, resulting in lower overall insulin levels. With lower insulin levels come lower LDL and triglyceride levels and higher HDL levels. With increased satiety comes lower caloric intake that leads to gradual weight normalization and improvements in blood pressure and a general sense of well-being over time. With improved bowel habits come reduced rates of diverticular disease. Fiber is good for you and you should get plenty of it (at least 25 grams per day). And fiber can only come in a carbohydrate package.

A carbohydrate-rich food is sufficiently high in fiber when it contains at least 2 grams of fiber per 100 calories.

I've noticed several items appearing on food shelves recently that boast very high fiber content. Although high fiber intake is good, getting all of your fiber in one sitting may not be the most beneficial dietary strategy. Fiber intake should be part of every meal; it should be spread out during the day. You want to realize the beneficial effects of fiber (slower food absorption, increased satiety, lower insulin levels) every time you eat. Just meeting your daily "fiber quota" with one bowl of cereal or one bar does not accomplish this. And a large dose of fiber all at once can lead to undesirable intestinal effects. Finally, a highly processed food product which has been fortified with fiber does not necessarily result in a healthful item. The simpler, the less complicated, the more "real" the food, the better it is for us. If we get back to the basics, we'll eat a higher fiber diet by default.

Ingredient #9: Eat your fruits and vegetables!

Nothing will benefit human health and increase the chances for survival of life on Earth as much as the evolution to a vegetarian diet.
— ALBERT EINSTEIN (1879–1955)

Your mother and grandmother were right! Eat plenty of fruits and vegetables every day. This rule is very simple and easy to follow — but we usually don't. The fruit and vegetable department is one place where you don't need to worry too much about moderation.

Here are a few things to remember:

- Raw is better than cooked
- Frozen is better than canned
- The less processed the better
- Choose the fruit not the juice

When I talk about fruits and vegetables, I mean fruits and vegetables. I don't mean French fries, ketchup, apple pie, or fruit jam. The more adulterated, processed and transformed the food, the less of it you should have. The more extras that come with it (canned peaches packed in heavy syrup, for example), the less healthy it is.

Fruits

The fourth point — choose the fruit not the juice — is an important one. Many people will enumerate how much fruit juice they consume, thinking they are being so good. I even had one patient tell me that he drank three to four *quarts* of orange juice a day because he thought this would be very healthy. Not surprisingly, he was tremendously overweight. Although fruit juice does contain many vitamins and minerals, it delivers these nutrients in a less fiber-full and higher calorie form. It takes several oranges to produce one large glass of orange juice — that's a lot of calories. You would be much better off eating the actual orange. The whole orange would be just as (or even more) satisfying than the glass of juice, would provide plenty of vitamins and minerals, and would pack a much higher fiber load per calorie consumed. If you can't see yourself giving up juice, try to drink it in reasonable quantities (remember — a serving is a half cup!) and dilute it with plenty of water.

For better taste and fewer chemicals and preservatives, choose locally grown, in-season, organic fruit. I personally favor buying local organic produce when I can, but eating plenty of fresh fruit every day is the point. If organic is available and affordable for you, choose organic. If organic is not available or not affordable, *eat plenty of fresh fruit every day anyway.*

Dried fruits are also fine. They have less vitamin C than do fresh fruits, but they still contain a lot of the beneficial antioxidants, fiber, and micronutrients found in fresh fruit. Dried fruits are more concentrated, so any pesticides and chemicals will be more likely to be concentrated as well. Here I would advise that you favor organic dried fruits whenever possible.

You should consume at least three fruit servings per day, and ideally five. *A serving of fresh fruit is* one-half cup of berries or cut-up fruit; one medium apple, orange, or banana; half of a grapefruit; three to four apricots; one large peach ... You get the idea. I'm basically describing a rough guide to a half-cup volume for each fruit (remember that tennis ball!). For dried fruit, think back to how much fruit would be in the fresh form and roughly calculate the dried equivalent. For apricots, it's easy: three fresh = three dried. Same for plums and prunes. For grapes and raisins, you're roughly talking 1/4 cup raisins for 1 cup grapes. Again, don't get too obsessed about food equivalents here — it's just fruit, for heaven's sake! And you can have whatever fruit you want, whenever you want. When was the last time you got a carte blanche invitation like that?

> *I don't care which fruit you consume, as long as you get some variety and get several servings a day — period.*

I am a big fan of berries — strawberries, blueberries, raspberries, cranberries. If there's "berry" in the name, I'm all over it! I love the taste of all these fruits, and I love the especially high concentrations of antioxidants in these little packages. Blueberries are my choice at breakfast. Cranberry relish is my favorite condiment. My older son loves pears, raspberries and bananas, and my younger son will gobble down mango, pineapple, or any melon I put in front of him. Neither will eat a cherry or ask for more papaya. My point? All fruits have value. Yes, some may be more packed with this, that, or the other — but the bottom line is *all fruit is good for you*. So remember to eat fruit several times a day. You need to consume at least 1½ cups of fresh fruit (or it's equivalent) every day.

You can be creative with fruit. Consider pureeing fruit with yogurt for breakfast — this is a healthy, "smoothie" way to start your day, especially if you sneak in a little flax meal, wheat germ, or a few walnuts. Think about baking some plain, fresh fruit under a thin cover of oat-based crunchy topping for a great dessert. Or just stick a bunch of fresh, peeled, cored and chilled pineapple into a blender and blend until frothy and smooth. Serve immediately with a couple of sliced up strawberries in a fancy wine glass for dessert. I guarantee you won't believe how phenomenally tasty and satisfying this dessert is! (I have actually served blended pineapple at the end of several of my formal dinner parties. My guests are always amazed at this dessert's delicious, simple, and decadent taste.)

Vegetables

When I say eat plenty of vegetables, I mean *all* vegetables. Yes, even the lowly potato. Many people stopped eating vegetables altogether when they got onto the high-protein bandwagon. Even though many vegetables are actually low carb, the difficulty in keeping track of which ones weren't made it easier just to quit eating all vegetables other than lettuce.

I don't think I've ever seen anyone consume as much lettuce with Caesar dressing as my husband did during his Atkins heyday (no croutons, of course). Tomatoes? Carrots? Too glycemic! Can't sabotage that 24-ounce steak by mixing in sugar! It does sound ridiculous now, doesn't it? But there's no denying it — the weight loss that some people realized with the high-protein plans overcame the commonsense notion that shying away from fruits and vegetables is simply not prudent for overall health.

You should think of vegetables as the *absolute foundation* of your diet. You should have more vegetables than fruit on any given day — five to seven servings of vegetables every day. A vegetable serving size is similar to that of fruit — one serving of fresh or cooked vegetables is ½ cup. For leafy greens, it's one cup. For vegetable juice, it's ½ cup. Unlike fruit juice, vegetable juice is relatively low in calories and simple sugars, so dilution is less critical. In fact, you could use vegetable juice to dilute fruit juice!

As with fruit, *you really can't eat too many vegetables*. Even though certain vegetables have more nutrients than do others, I don't care which ones you eat as long as you're eating a variety of vegetables several times a day.

Variety is key, though: If your five servings of vegetables are all potatoes (or other starchy varieties like corn), you could be setting yourself up for easier weight gain by stimulating more of that insulin release, which pushes your metabolism into storage mode. And remember — a serving is a half cup — that's about half of a typical baked potato. For starchier vegetables, watching portion size *is* important. And I would not eat starchy vegetables every day.

The other key is to serve your vegetables as simply as possible. Once you start dousing your broccoli with cheese sauce you've pretty much left the vegetable category behind. On that baked potato, favor chives and herbs and go easy on the butter.

Now, my earlier quip about lettuce does not mean you should shy away from it. Eating salads is a wonderful way of ensuring that you meet your vegetable quotient. The more colorful your salad the better! Sprinkling sunflower seeds or nuts on top can really turn a salad into something more substantial and filling. Add a lean protein source (grilled fish, chicken, hard-boiled eggs) and you have a meal. For dressings, choose vinaigrettes and avoid mayonnaise-based sauces. Always ask for the dressing on the side — I guarantee you will use less of it than you would if it's poured all over the salad for you. Dip your fork into the dressing before you dip your fork into the salad. This is a great way to ensure getting the dressing's taste with every mouthful.

Here's a general rule to follow:

When assembling the components of your lunch or dinner, start by planning your vegetables first.

Think about the three vegetable servings you need to accommodate in that meal. We make a mistake when we start with the protein and build the meal around that. Work backwards. Start with the veggies and then worry about the protein. Be creative and daring. Experiment with vegetables you haven't tried before. Favor raw or steamed preparations. Sautéing fresh vegetables in a little bit of olive oil is also an excellent preparation. Sprinkle those sautéed vegetables with some herbs and lemon juice — now you're singing!

Don't forget about soups — they're fabulous vehicles for incorporating vegetables into your day. Think minestrone, chicken vegetable, tomato ... but make sure they're broth based, please. If you crave creamy soups, consider adding a cooked potato and puréeing, or start off the soup with vegetables especially good for blending (squash, pumpkin, celery root, etc. — even peppers and carrots). I consider a soup and salad the perfect dinner or lunch. When the soup contains some whole grains (barley, brown or wild rice, etc.) and protein (chicken, turkey, lean beef, tofu, fish), you have a truly filling and satisfying meal on your hands (and in your stomach).

Beans and legumes

One very important food category fits loosely in the fruit and vegetable section: beans and legumes. Beans and legumes are especially good food choices — full of fiber, folate, *and* protein, making them a great substitute for meats. A serving of beans or legumes is ½ cup cooked. You can use one serving of legumes to cover both a protein/meat serving as well as one vegetable serving in one fell swoop. My favorite appetizer? Hummus (heavy on the garlic!) with raw vegetables. My favorite winter-time meal? Vegetarian chili — with lots of cilantro!

> *Fruits and vegetables, beans and legumes — these need to be the foundation of your nutritional plan. Believe me, you will be way ahead of the game if you become best friends with the produce section!*

Ingredient #10: Choose smart fat, not low fat

Many people believe that the fastest way to a better cholesterol profile and a smaller waistline is by eliminating fat from their diets. Actually nothing could be further from the truth. Fat is not directly related to the cholesterol numbers and we need a certain amount of fat in our diets for optimal health. Just as with carbohydrates, however, there are good fats and bad fats, and moderation is still key.

Saturated fats

The fats you should limit in your diet are **saturated fats**. These are the fats that are solid at room temperature: butter, shortening, lard, fatty milk or cream, cheese, the marbling in beef and the fat in chicken are the most common examples. These are all fats that tend to raise LDL cholesterol levels. But you can't completely avoid these foods, nor should you have to. We're back to that balance thing. And if you want to know the truth — I love cheese. I can't imagine a world without cheese. I also can't imagine eating bread without butter or never having another steak.

But I don't eat steak every day. And when I do, I usually have a small filet and cut off any fatty portions. I eat bread with butter, but I only put the butter on when it will make a difference to the taste (and that's actually not all that often). I eat cheese, but I try to eat it in reasonable amounts and try to balance the calories and fat from it by not going crazy with other high-calorie ingredients and foods at the same sitting. And I stop eating when I'm full.

What should your strategy be? When you eat beef, eat a smaller portion and remove any visible fat. Think of the beef as your side dish and make the vegetables the main part of the meal. You'll still get all the taste of the food you love, but you'll just eat it in a different proportion. When you're out at a steakhouse, don't order the biggest cut you can — order the most flavorful and highest quality.

When you're eating chicken, don't eat the skin and do cut off all the visible fat. Just as with beef, eat a smaller portion. Also pay attention to what else lands on your plate. If you're already eating beef or chicken, consuming a heavy accompaniment (like scalloped potatoes) makes no sense. Balance the dicey food choices with a more healthful array of sides: steamed vegetables, a salad, fruit for dessert. This is actually not all that complicated.

Stay true to portion control! A serving size of meat is three ounces. I had always felt so restrained when I ordered the six-ounce petite filet at our favorite steakhouse, especially compared to the 16-ounce sirloin or the 24-ounce (!) porterhouse choices. But I was actually eating enough meat for two people; and that 24-ounce steak is enough meat for a family of eight!

In the ideal world, you should be consuming zero to three portions of animal protein per day to ensure you are avoiding the bad fats. So really, your absolute maximum for that steak should be eight ounces (with no other meats or animal protein the rest of the day). You can be much less restrictive with fish portions, but you still need to be within reasonable limits from a calorie perspective. Eating fish at least twice per week should be your goal. Favoring vegetarian protein is a good strategy (a portion of vegetarian protein would be one egg, or two egg whites, or three ounces of tofu, or ½ cup cooked beans or legumes). Three to six portions of vegetarian protein per day is fine.

Nonsaturated fats

The fats you don't need to worry about or actively limit are the **nonsaturated fats** — those that remain liquid at room temperature. Olive oil, canola oil, the oils in nuts and seeds, the oils in avocados and fish ... These are all healthful and actually help boost HDL cholesterol while helping reduce LDL and triglycerides.

Fish oils (which contain an abundance of omega-3 fatty acids in the DHA and EPA forms) are especially healthful. People who consume fish regularly display lower rates of cardiovascular disease and stroke. Recently, fish consumption has been linked to lower levels of inflammatory markers (that C-reactive protein we talked about earlier) in the blood. But be careful about how you prepare that fish. Grilling, broiling, or steaming is good; frying or sautéing is bad. *The guiding principles are the same as for fruits and vegetables — the less processed or altered the better.* When you serve fish, think about how it might be served in a Mediterranean country — freshly caught, simply prepared, unadorned by too many sides or other taste distractions. My favorite fish? Salmon. It's full of omega fatty acids and natural antioxidants. My mouth is watering just writing about it!

What about mercury? Just when you think you have the perfect food, it has to get gummed up by toxins. Yes, mercury is a concern and some fish have higher contents than do others. Mackerel and swordfish are known to be especially vulnerable to higher-than-desirable levels of this contaminant. Restrict your intake of these fish: Eat no more than one serving per week generally, and no servings for pregnant women. Other fish are by and large fine. Your strategy should be to eat fewer servings of the huge fish at the top of the food chain, since toxins are more likely to be concentrated in them. (I would put tuna in this category even though tuna is high in omega-3 fatty acids.)

For those of you who absolutely, positively, no way, no how, will eat fish, consider incorporating flaxseed oil or flax meal into your life. Flax oil also provides omega-3 fatty acids and has similar effects on the lipid profile as do fish oils. The omega-3 fatty acid found in flax (and nuts) is ALA, a slightly different form than the omega-3 found in fish. It first has to be metabolized within our bodies to be effective, so this is a somewhat less efficient way to obtain omega-3s than eating fish — but it is still very healthful. You can use flaxseed oil as a substitute for olive oil in your salad dressing. You can find flaxseed oil in many supermarkets and health food stores in a refrigerated case in an opaque container. Flax meal also provides omega-3 fatty acids, which is why it is an excellent fiber supplement for cereal or when baking bread. Flax seeds themselves are a less useful item because we can't digest the seeds very well, and could therefore miss out on the nutritional benefits of the flax core. If you buy flax seeds, you should grind them before eating.

Go nuts

What about nuts? Nuts are a very healthful food group, offering high protein content packaged with beneficial fats (including those omegas). I consider nuts to be a wonderful food on their own, and something worth adding to other foods to boost nutritional content and increase satiety. But nuts are high in calories, so we have to remember the calories in versus calories out principle. As healthy as they may be, consuming a jar of nuts is simply not reasonable. A single serving of almonds is about 24 whole nuts; a single serving of walnuts is about 15 walnut halves. Keeping your nut consumption to a handful or so per day is acceptable. Avoiding processed nuts is a must. The more "handled" the nut, the lower the overall nutritional value. So avoid salted, honeyed and the various flavored nuts and instead favor raw nuts. Raw walnuts, raw almonds and raw sunflower seeds are especially good choices. If you need to snack, try substituting a few raw walnuts for that bag of chips or candy bar. Your heart will thank you for it.

Trans fats

Trans fats are artificially modified fats used to enhance the texture, taste, and shelf life of many processed foods. Trans fats are especially adroit at messing with your cholesterol profile: Eating them not only raises LDL levels but also lowers HDL levels. They have no set safe limit for consumption and should be avoided altogether. How do you avoid trans fats? By avoiding processed foods — especially fast food, mass-produced bakery-type items (think cookies, rolls and cakes), and snack foods (like chips and many crackers). When in doubt, check the label. If you see the item containing *any* trans fat (usually listed as hydrogenated or partially hydrogenated fats), think long and hard before deciding to put it in your mouth. Trans fats are about as far as you can get from smart fats.

Omega-3s

Unlike the advice for trans fats, we should be actively incorporating omega-3s into our diet. Ideally, we should all be obtaining, on average, at least one gram of omega-3 fatty acids on a daily basis, and even up to three grams per day. As mentioned above, good dietary sources of omega-3 fatty acids include oily fish (like salmon and herring), walnuts, and flax meal/oil. Three ounces (that's a pretty small portion!) of salmon contains about one and one-half grams of omega-3. One tablespoon of flax seed oil will provide about one gram of biologically active omega-3s.

Don't confuse comega-3s with omega-6 fatty acids. These do not confer the same health benefits as omega-3s — so when you're evaluating food composition, just concentrate on omega-3 content.

As we now know, the easiest way of obtaining beneficial omega-3s is by eating more fish. But not all fish is created equal. Beware of fast food fish items and the frozen convenience-type fried fish products. These are all relatively low in omega-3s and high in trans fats. The best choice (broken record here!) is a small- to medium-sized portion of fresh fish, prepared simply and served without too many adornments.

If you don't like fish, taking a fish oil supplement is not a bad idea. Depending on the preparation, up to three (or more!) fish oil capsules per day may be required to provide the one gram per day of omega-3 fatty acids. Check the label of the supplement for total milligrams of EPA and DHA (omega-3s) in each tablet to figure out how many tablets a day you need to get to the one gram total.

Some people will notice a fishy aftertaste with omega-3 or fish-oil supplementation. In large doses (over three gm/day), stomach upset is possible. In patients with metabolic syndrome or high triglycerides, a rise in LDL levels is possible with high doses of omega-3. In diabetics, worsening blood sugar control is also possible with very high omega-3-fatty-acid supplementation. It's always a good idea to review your supplement intake with your physician.

Ingredient #11: Allow an egg a day (don't obsess over the cholesterol)

Eggs are full of cholesterol, right? So they must be bad, right?

Here's a rule that actually lets you off the hook a bit! Although many scientific bodies recommend limiting cholesterol intake, I don't find that counting cholesterol grams is all that useful from a practical perspective. For example, plenty of cookies carry the "low cholesterol" label. But I would argue that even if it's low in cholesterol that cookie is not very healthful. I find that the cholesterol content is secondary: If you make wise fat choices and wise carbohydrate choices, you will be making good cholesterol choices by default. So a low-saturated-fat, low-sugar, high-fiber cookie (OK, they don't exist) will be naturally low in cholesterol: You get the point!

Another fact that lowers the importance of cholesterol counting in my mind is that some foods that are relatively high in cholesterol are actually quite healthful — foods like shrimp, lobster, and so forth. These seafood items are very high in protein and low in fat, and relatively low in calories. Cholesterol in these food items therefore has much less of a negative effect on your biochemistry. Now, smothering the shrimp or lobster with a butter-based sauce will dramatically change the health effect of that shrimp or lobster. All of a sudden you will be ingesting the cholesterol with a bunch of saturated fat — and that's not ideal. In fact, as far as your body is concerned, you will have basically changed a healthful seafood choice into a piece of fatty steak. So it's not the cholesterol, it's what it's traveling with that's important.

Eggs are fine. I see nothing wrong with eating an egg or two a day. For their nutritional value, eggs are an excellent food source. The egg yolk contains some saturated fat (so going overboard is not wise), but I never discourage egg intake. I'd rather see someone eat a couple of eggs than a stack of regular pancakes any day.

Also keep in mind that our bodies manufacture the vast majority of the cholesterol in our bloodstream, so the cholesterol we consume accounts for only a tiny fraction of what's actually circulating in our system. The type and amount of cholesterol you make is influenced more by your dietary fat and carbohydrate choices — and your genetics — than by the cholesterol content of food. So concentrate on limiting saturated fat and simple carbohydrates; everything else will fall in line.

Occasionally, when a patient's blood cholesterol levels are borderline for requiring treatment or increasing medications, I will go over cholesterol consumption with him or her and, if appropriate, have that person cut out some of the higher cholesterol choices they are consuming to see whether this makes a difference. This situation occurs infrequently in my practice, and it is the rare individual who already eats a healthful diet from the carbohydrate and fat perspective who realizes a significant change in his or her profile by not eating an egg or two. *It really is the overall diet balance that determines your cholesterol numbers* (above and beyond your genetic makeup, weight, and activity level).

Ingredient #12: Put down the salt shaker

Some people consume amazing quantities of salt. Just as we have to readjust our sweet meters, we need to revamp our salt habits. In terms of our daily needs for sodium, we would get enough of this mineral if we ate all of our food without ever adding a single grain of salt during preparation. In other words, *adequate salt is no added salt at all.* So every grain of salt from the shaker is salt we don't really need. That's a pretty sobering baseline. On the other hand, I'll be the first to admit that a diet completely devoid of any added salt can be somewhat dull on the taste buds. It's not realistic for me to advise you to never use salt again. But it is realistic for me to ask you to examine how and when you add salt to your foods.

Add salt to my foods? I find that the food I buy is salty enough already. I don't even have a salt shaker on the table. Aha! Gotcha! If you are consuming foods that are processed, canned, or preprepared (including partially premade foods that you complete at home), chances are good that you are consuming a boatload of sodium even if you don't add any more salt at the table. So if you can, try to avoid these items, or at least choose low-sodium alternatives.

If you love soup, and find yourself eating canned versions, consider making a large pot of soup from scratch and freezing smaller portions in sealed plastic bags for another time. Yes, this involves some effort (but not that much). Doesn't your body deserve it? If you love the convenience of canned vegetables, consider switching to fresh frozen. They are just as easy to prepare, contain no added salt, and are significantly more nutritious. If you eat at fast food restaurants — *stop!* (It's not just the sodium that's an issue here.) And if you eat out often, avoid sprinkling extra salt on your food and consider asking that your food be prepared without added salt or with reduced salt content.

Another strategy for reducing salt intake while maintaining flavor is to use herbs in cooking. These days, our supermarkets stock dried and fresh herbs year round in a wide array of choices. Experiment beyond parsley and chives. Basil is a perfect partner for tomatoes or any Italian-inspired dish. Oregano is perfect with chicken or olives. Sage is wonderful with pork. Rosemary goes with hearty stews and meats. Tarragon is fabulous with egg dishes. And thyme and dill work great with fish. This is just the tip of the iceberg. Experiment with herbs; learn to mix and match. Think about starting a small herb garden either outdoors or on your windowsill. Enjoy the aroma and taste sensation that these little additions bring to your food. You'll find that as you use more herbs, you will need less salt.

Ingredient #13: Make food special

In our fast-paced world, we tend to gulp our food on the go. The faster, the more convenient, the better. We eat in front of the television set and the computer screen. We eat standing up in our kitchens. We eat in our cars. We have no set mealtimes and no set menus. We don't really spend much time or invest much effort in tasting the food. And when we have no ceremony around food consumption, it becomes very easy to lose track of when we're consuming, how much we're consuming, and what we're consuming.

Setting a predetermined time for eating puts the breaks on eating at other times.

I personally believe that the disappearance of the rituals that used to surround eating has contributed in a major way to the obesity epidemic. Setting a predetermined time for eating puts the breaks on eating at other times. And it helps to put preparing and eating food back on center stage as more of an event, rather than a side activity. When we give food more attention, we can concentrate on quality, quantity, and nutritional value.

Growing up, I always had dinner at 5:30 p.m. My whole family gathered at the table for a home-cooked meal. We always had soup, then some sort of main course and always dessert (from my mom's bakery, of course). It wasn't a big, drawn-out event — sometimes it lasted all of 15 minutes with the meal consumed in silence — but we always knew that come hell or high water we were to be at that table together at 5:30 p.m. There was something special about that routine.

I find sitting down to a regular meal at 5:30 p.m. laughable today — I'm just starting to wind down my workday at that time! I make the effort to gather everyone at 7 p.m. around our kitchen table for a meal, with the table set and a prayerful thanks to start us off. Sometimes it's just soup, sometimes it's leftovers (again!). Sometimes we don't actually sit down until 8 p.m. But the sense of routine and stability is priceless. And the nutritional value and food quality are under my control.

So make food consumption special! Establish a schedule for meals. It may not work every day to set the table with the good china, or even expect everyone to show up at the table on time. But try to make eating more ritualistic, with a bit more pomp and circumstance. When you devote all that extra attention, you'll find it harder to waste it on junk.

Ingredient #14: Prepare your own food

The most remarkable thing about my mother is that for thirty years she served the family nothing but leftovers. The original meal has never been found.
— CALVIN TRILLIN

I've slipped it in here and there, but now I'm about to say it directly: You have to start making some of your food. No, I don't mean harvesting the wheat and making the flour. I mean cooking. And not just opening a can or a box of ingredients. I mean cooking from scratch: making a stew, baking some fresh fish, chopping some vegetables. It doesn't have to be fancy or complicated. It just has to be made by *you*.

Ultimately, food you cook is food you have complete control over. *You* decide the fat source. *You* decide on the amount of salt. *You* decide the fiber content. If you've never cooked before, start with something easy — boil an egg. Get good at making salads or cooking soups. Ask a relative or a friend for a cooking lesson. But get cooking!

If we interact more with our food, we'll elevate our experience and expectations, and poor choices will be easier to spot and easier to avoid.

Many cookbooks on the market today target the health-conscious chef. Browse the shelves of your local library or bookstore and see what appeals to you. Cooking magazines and cooking shows may provide inspiration as well. Regardless of your recipe sources, you will enjoy many benefits from a more intimate relationship with your food.

Ingredient #15: Never ever eat fast food

It doesn't take watching the film "Supersize Me" to know that fast food is bad for us. If you haven't seen this movie, I highly recommend that you do. It's sobering indeed to see how quickly the calories and fat from fast food exert their effects. Fast food is the food you have the least control over. And it is most likely to be of worst quality and highest in sugar, salt, and fat content.

You buy it on impulse (usually when you're hungry), letting your eyes (not your stomach) guide your choices. You eat the food quickly, often after driving past the pick-up window. And you miss out on the meal planning and anticipation, the meal experience, and the nutritional value of food. Your body can take getting beat up like this only so many times before your health is affected. Don't give in to the attractive signs and the "good deals." Your health and your heart are way too valuable to be squandered away like this.

Due to external pressures, some fast food restaurants are beginning to offer more healthful (or at least healthful-sounding) choices on their menus. But just because the deep-fried piece of chicken meat now comes with lettuce and dressing doesn't mean it's necessarily better for you or less caloric than if it came sandwiched in a bun. Keep your guard up. *Your basic strategy is still to eat less processed food, reduce your intake of saturated fat and simple starches, and increase your intake of fiber*. Don't forget these rules if you order a meal in a fast food establishment.

One advantage you have is that most fast food restaurants and chains now offer information regarding the nutritional content of their menu items — if not in the restaurant, then at least on their Web sites. Check that information before ordering your food. You might be surprised which items turn out to be the big no-no's!

Ingredient #16: Choose your fluids wisely

Water is the most neglected nutrient in your diet
but one of the most vital.
— KELLY BARTON

When I go over dietary habits with my patients, I always make sure to also ask them about what they drink — and I'm not just asking about alcohol consumption. I'm often surprised at the amounts of soda, juice, and other high-calorie beverages people consume. This can be the most obvious and easy place to modify your diet if you are overweight. By changing from sugared and high-calorie beverages to water and diet beverages you can shave off an incredible number of calories from your intake without much sacrifice.

Fruit juice

But if you want to aim for living as healthfully as possible, go one step further and make water your beverage of choice. Juice? Well, remember the rule from Ingredient #9: Choose the fruit not the juice. But if you or your children continue to drink juice, decrease the frequency and volume (one serving is a *half cup*), and always dilute the juice with water. To start, you might want to just add a small amount of water and increase the proportion over time. Your goal should be to get to a mixture where water makes up at least half of the beverage. Eventually, you will notice that an undiluted serving of juice will be unpalatably sweet and overly filling. And by always diluting juice for children, you can influence their drinking habits for the long haul and change their palates toward less sweet and less simple-carbohydrate-type food choices.

Hot beverages

For hot beverages, choose tea over coffee, not because coffee is necessarily harmful or causes heart disease but because tea appears to be more healthful. Green tea especially is full of antioxidants and appears to have multiple health benefits. Herbal teas? They're OK, but on balance not nearly as antioxidant-full as green or regular black tea. If you are trying to avoid caffeine, herbal tea is definitely the way to go (even decaffeinated tea and coffee still have some caffeine in them).

Ingredient #17: A calorie is *not* a calorie is *not* a calorie

> ***Tell me what you eat***
> ***and I will tell you what you are.***
> — Anthelme Brillat-Savarin (1755–1826)

You know what I said earlier about a calorie being a calorie being a calorie? Well, that's only partially true. It definitely applies to weight loss — energywise, you have to balance what goes in and what goes out. But from a health perspective not all calories are created equal. The 300 calories from a candy bar have nowhere near the nutritional value of 300 calories from a small piece of grilled salmon and a salad.

> *Remember: Whatever you put in your mouth has to be*
> *processed by your body. Garbage in truly equals garbage out.*

It's really important that you make a conscious effort to eat only high-quality foods in reasonable amounts. That's really the bottom line, and is the real recipe for healthy eating. These foods are not exotic or complicated. They're not even necessarily expensive. Fruits and vegetables, high-fiber grains, beans and legumes, fish and raw nuts, tea. If your diet favors these ingredients, you will be ahead of the game. Even if nothing happens to your cholesterol profile because you have changed your eating habits, you will still be healthier and at lower risk of developing heart disease.

You *always* have a choice as to what you put or don't put in your mouth. Do your best to always make the right choice.

Food for thought

Your diet is not just a critical component of your heart health, but of your complete lifestyle. This chapter's principal guidance can be summarized as —

- Choose your foods wisely. Garbage in equals garbage out. Don't be a trash can.

- Consume food in reasonable quantities. Portion control is weight control.

- Enjoy a wide variety of foods from every food category. Deprivation does not work. But this does not cancel out the first rule — junk is junk is junk and you should not eat it.

- Increase your intake of fruits and vegetables. Raw! Raw! Raw!

- Add beans and legumes to your diet as a substitute for meat and to add fiber.

- Choose water and tea as beverages. Dilute all fruit juices with water.

- Start preparing more of your food. Control is power.

- Unless you're a grazer, growing, or an athlete — stop snacking.

- Balance any obvious indiscretions.

- Remember to savor and enjoy your food — stop fighting with it!

Piece of Advice #13

If you're having trouble sticking with good food habits,
try this visualization aid: Imagine you own the car of your
dreams — a Ferrari, a Bentley, a Porsche ... whatever really
tickles your fancy. Now imagine that the car manual calls
for using only premium unleaded fuel to fill the gas tank. Would
you then go and use diesel? Why, you wouldn't dream of it! So why
would you *ever* use the wrong fuel to fill your body? Your body is far
more complex, sophisticated, and valuable than any car. Use only
the recommended fuels to keep it in the best possible condition.
Treat your body as if it were a Ferrari! (And while you're at it, take it
out for a spin.)

Everything counts

Everything you put in is processed by your body. So if you pick up the
wrong fuel pump and start putting the wrong gas into your Ferrari, don't
just keep filling the tank! Rectify your mistakes as quickly as possible.

Good nutrition is a commitment. It might take you a few months to get to
a healthful eating regimen for every meal. That's OK. As long as you're making
positive changes, you're getting healthier and your heart is getting happier.

Finally, if you are overweight, remember that you didn't get to your
present weight overnight, so expecting to get down to your ideal weight
instantly is just not realistic. Long-term weight control involves long-term,
healthy eating habits. If you follow the advice in this chapter, you might not
drop pounds like rocks, but over time you *will* get to your healthy weight
and be much more likely to stay slim for the long haul.

And don't lose sight of this fact: Your actions at the supermarket and at the restaurant do have far-reaching effects. By being a wiser consumer, you will send a signal to your food and nutrient suppliers — and they listen very intently. They simply want to make what sells. If you signal a change in buying habits, they will respond by changing the product choices. As consumers, we have the power to alter the food landscape in front of us, not by yelling and demanding, but by whispering through our pocketbooks.

Visit __www.CardioSmart.org__ for tips and tools to help you take control and make smart food choices

CHAPTER 16

Move Your Groove Thing

Walking is the best possible exercise.
Habituate yourself to walk very far.
— THOMAS JEFFERSON (1743–1826)

"I can't believe it started."

"It's been sitting here in this parking lot for months, but one turn of the engine and it started up!"

"I just can't believe it started!"

My husband and I go through this same routine at least three times a year. We keep an old car at one of the Denver airport's park-and-fly lots. Between our visits to the mountains, the car sits there for months at a time in the middle of an asphalt plain. As the airport shuttle brings us to our vehicle, we always wonder: Will it start?

A cornerstone of health

Just as it's not the best maintenance schedule to let your car sit for months at a time, your own best maintenance schedule doesn't entail your sitting around. A car needs to be driven and your body needs to move. Just as the chances of starting the car decrease the longer it sits idle, the chances of developing health problems increase the longer you remain sedentary. And it's not just the engine (heart) we're talking about here. Remember how you are going to feed your body like you would fuel a Ferrari? What good is owning the Ferrari if you don't drive it as often as you can?

Exercise is a cornerstone of every healthy lifestyle. And it has far-reaching benefits beyond heart-disease prevention. Being fit allows us to withstand events that might otherwise stop us in our tracks. I'm constantly amazed at how much more resilient fit people are when faced with any sort of illness. Just think of Lance Armstrong and his incredible comeback from metastatic cancer. By being exceptionally fit when diagnosed with his illness, he was able to tolerate and rebound from intense chemotherapy and surgery much better and more quickly than he would have had he been an overweight couch potato. And he rebounded to the pinnacle of human endurance!

Intriguing data are also emerging that exercise may have beneficial effects on our metabolism, above and beyond mere calorie expenditure. It turns out that stress on our bones (from walking, for example), stimulates the production of osteocalcin (UH-stee-oh-KAL-sin), a hormone that promotes calcium deposition in bone (a good thing, because more calcium means a stronger skeletal system). As it turns out, osteocalcin also makes our cells more responsive to any insulin that is around, reducing the amount of insulin that has to circulate in our bloodstreams. And by now you should know well that lower insulin levels are generally beneficial, resulting in lower LDL and triglyceride levels, higher HDL numbers, and generally less efficient calorie hoarding. This last part may explain why individuals who have succeeded in losing weight and keeping it off are almost always those individuals who commenced and continued an exercise regimen in conjunction with altering their food intake. Bottom line? Exercise is good for you, for all sorts of reasons.

How much exercise?

The latest recommendations advise 60 to 90 minutes of exercise *every day*. I know; this seems unattainable to me, too. I can't fathom spending 60 minutes, let alone 90, on my treadmill every day (though that would be child's play for Mr. Armstrong!). What I *can* envision is spending 30 to 45 minutes in a warm-up/exercise/cool-down/stretch routine and increasing my activity in general during the day; so that I at least get close to that 60- to 90-minute recommendation. I might not increase my endurance as much by breaking up the workout, but I will still be burning calories and enhancing my overall health.

What do I mean by increasing activity in general? I mean adding movement to my day in bits and pieces. For example, rather than taking the elevator I might climb a flight of stairs or two (or three or four). And I always walk down the stairs. Typically, I will take a parking spot that's not the nearest to the store (although I admit that I don't take one that's farthest away either; there is some enjoyment in the "hunt"). I might turn on music when I'm making dinner and dance around the kitchen a little — occasionally I'll get my kids to join in. Yes, we look silly, but we sure have fun!

Love to burn

Exercise is a vital component of a healthy existence. It needs to be as much a part of your day as brushing your teeth or eating a meal. Here's how to make it happen —

- Thirty minutes of daily exercise is the *minimum*. We should be aiming to move our bodies for 60 to 90 minutes per day.

- If the minimum is too much right now, do what you can. It all counts.

- Longer periods of exercise are more beneficial for building endurance and are more likely to improve your fitness level than are shorter periods.

- If you can't devote longer periods during the day, incorporating 30 to 90 minutes of movement divided into small chunks is still beneficial because of the increased calorie expenditure.

- Enjoy a mix of activities that allow for both aerobic training and muscle building. Avoid doing muscle building as your *only* workout regimen.

- Establish an environment friendly to outdoor play for your children. Get outside yourself and get active with them. Imprint healthful habits as early as possible.

Weight management is all about calories in versus calories out. Burn baby burn!

People always ask me which exercise is best. My reply: whatever you like, as long as you move your body through space for at least a portion of the workout. In general, activities that principally involve muscle building (like weight lifting) are less beneficial from a cardiovascular perspective. But having strong, lean muscles is a good thing from a general health perspective, so weight training should definitely constitute a component of your regime. Muscular bodies also burn calories faster. However, concentrating exclusively on muscle building is not a balanced exercise strategy, just like eating only protein or only carbohydrates is not a balanced dietary strategy.

Walking

I like to see my patients do something aerobic every day (or most days of the week). I often recommend walking to patients who are not already committed to a particular workout regime. Walking is a wonderful form of exercise because it can be done almost anywhere and doesn't involve a lot of investment in expensive equipment. And you can incorporate it into your day relatively easily. If the weather is nice, consider using half of your lunch hour to go for a walk. Take a friend. Make it fun. If you have a dog, try to spend at least a half hour on a walk with it every day. This is as much about your health and well-being as it is about your pet's health and elimination schedule.

The fifteen-minute mile

In general, if you choose walking as one of your exercise activities, you should aim to walk at least two miles in half an hour. That means you are walking at a pretty good clip — four miles per hour. That's definitely slower than running, but it's also significantly faster than window-shopping speed or strolling. If you are a total couch potato when starting out, you could get to the two-miles-in-a-half-hour goal a couple of different ways. You could walk for a half hour every day and gradually increase the distance so that in that half hour you eventually cover two miles, or you could walk two miles each day and try to do it faster and faster each time until you manage to cover the distance in a half hour. Depending upon your lifestyle and other commitments, one of these approaches will be more viable for you.

If you walk on a treadmill, it's pretty easy to figure out when you covered two miles — the machine tells you. If you walk outdoors, you might need to measure your route by driving it first.

Regardless of the way you cover those two miles, you will have burned about 100 calories per mile. Whether you walk or run two miles, it's still about 100 calories per mile. Calorie expenditure is more a function of distance than of speed — you just burn the 100 calories faster if you run.

It all counts!

But what if what I'm describing sounds too difficult to attain right now, if two miles seem like a mountain and not a hill, if you literally do *no* exercise right now? Just start doing something — anything! Walk to the end of your driveway and back. Do a couple of laps around your dining table or your kitchen island. It all counts! Every step makes a difference. Every minute you don't spend sitting on your couch or at your desk is a minute of happiness for your heart.

For those individuals with a disability, physical activity, even if modest, is still very important. Follow the advice provided by your physical therapist or physician. Although becoming very fit may not be a reasonable goal, maintaining and improving strength and flexibility through customized exercises is critical for your overall health.

And just to emphasize again, exercise has many benefits beyond weight loss. People who exercise regularly sleep better, are more relaxed and generally experience higher self-esteem. Fitness breeds fitness. The more active you are the more active you want to be. This is a positive, self-perpetuating cycle — and there aren't that many of those!

So ... Get moving. If you're already exercising on a regular basis, keep going! If you're just starting, set reasonable goals and keep tabs on your progress. You would be well served to speak with your physician about your plans, to go over your exercise routine and establish a framework within which to achieve your goals. Always check with your physician before starting a new or significantly more strenuous activity pattern.

Make exercise and activity an integral part of your life. Incorporate it into other facets of your day. Exercise should be as much a part of your routine as brushing your teeth or getting dressed.

Active children

If you have young children, go walking with them and rediscover the world through their eyes. Play tag in the yard. Throw a ball around. Ride a bike. Teach them early to keep active so they stay active as they grow.

I believe that one of the reasons our children are becoming overweight is that they no longer play outside. They are either shuttled around to various activities or sitting in front of a television or computer screen. The seemingly unsupervised outdoor exploration that we all enjoyed as children is not part of the plans for our offspring.

When was the last time you let your child take off on a bike in the morning, not expecting to see them again until dinner? For safety reasons, we no longer feel comfortable letting our children play outside by themselves. So we drive them to sports practice and cheer them on, drive past a pick-up window to pick up food (since we no longer have time to make the meal), and then have them sit inside the house enjoying the latest video game while we work longer and longer hours to pay for the sports activities, takeout meals, and computers. We've gotten ourselves caught in a time-and-money trap, and our children are the casualties.

What if *we* were outside with our children? Imagine if all your neighbors were physically active, if they took time to go for walks or work in their gardens. All of a sudden you would have a readymade neighborhood-watch program on your hands. And your children could be outside because all your neighbors would be out there too. Instead of driving them to activities, what if you just encouraged your children to play with other kids in the neighborhood and then just hung out around your house? What if your neighbors did the same? We might just get back to that time when going outside to explore or ride a bike was *normal.*

We have become an increasingly insular and isolated society. And our children's health has suffered because of this. It's time for us to be a bit more neighborly and more physically active. Let's get our children outdoors — they won't think of it as exercise or a strategy to balance calorie intake. They'll just remember the time they discovered an anthill in your neighbor's yard, or the first time they did a wheelie with the kids down the block.

Active adults

Back to adults ... I often have patients tell me they have no time to add exercise to their busy schedules. But when we go over what they do during the day, we end up finding opportunities to add movement. One of the easiest recommendations is to have patients exercise while they participate in another activity. If you spend time watching television or listening to music, incorporate movement into those times. Maybe you need to park a stationary bike or a treadmill in front of the television screen. But don't leave it in park! If you play golf, walk the course instead of riding the cart. If you read for pleasure, think about listening to books on tape while going for a walk.

Travel

If you travel for business (or for pleasure), take advantage of your hotel's workout facilities. Plan for that by always packing some running shoes, shorts, and a T-shirt whenever you're going out of town. Then make sure you save some time for yourself while on the road. Use exercise and activity to recharge, regenerate and refocus. If you have the choice on your vacations, opt for walking tours and other sightseeing activities that include some physical exercise. Add physical activity in small increments whenever you can. You know what they say: Ten thousand steps a day keeps the doctor away! (You can purchase a pedometer and keep track of the steps you take. Aim to exceed that 10,000 mark every day.)

Time constraints

Sometimes, when my patients and I examine their schedules, we really do come up against time constraints. Their days are completely filled with responsibilities and activities, usually work related. Under these circumstances patients are often stressed and exhausted and simply collapse at the end of their days. My advice here is usually met with skepticism, but almost always works out well. I tell those patients to add exercise anyway. Even if it means waking up earlier (yes, even if it's at 5 a.m. or before) or going to bed later, I advise them to add exercise to their day. Most patients find that over time, they actually have more energy and become more efficient during their other tasks. In fact, their days often *shorten* in the long haul and they feel dramatically better over time. Taking that 30 minutes to one hour every day also gives those people a little time to reflect on their circumstances and to prioritize their activities and responsibilities during the rest of the day. Sometimes this results in reorganization and reprioritization, leading to positive changes, like more realistic work schedules and saner existences.

Buddy up

Some people do better when they establish a buddy system. The idea that you might let someone else down if you don't show up or if you don't pull your own weight can really motivate certain people. If this is you, plan regular times to exercise with a friend or your spouse. Committing to a personal trainer falls into this same category and may be the solution for some. *Regardless of your approach or motivation, you must exercise. You must move your body.*

Only *you* can exercise your body. No one else can do this for you. There are no pills you can take or special equipment you can buy that will substitute for your own physical effort.

So, move your groove thing! (And if you pull out the disco ball, I'm there!)

Piece of Advice # 14

Think of exercise as a payment to yourself. One of the best pieces of advice I ever got about saving money was to always pay myself first before I paid any other bills. This ensured that I put away a little money every month, and pretty soon that "little money" began to add up. If I had never paid myself, that money would have been spent on "stuff" and my savings would have been nonexistent. If you don't make a commitment to save, you will never get ahead in creating wealth. Make exercise a priority payment that you make to yourself every day. There will always be other ways to "spend" your time — but unless you "pay" yourself first, you will never get ahead in creating health.

CHAPTER 17

A Spitting Image

We are survival machines —
robot vehicles blindly programmed to preserve
the selfish molecules known as genes.
— RICHARD DAWKINS

D o you remember the story about the three little pigs? One little pig built his house out of straw, one built his house out of sticks, and one used bricks. I bet you never knew that this story was really about genetics!

Same genes, different health

Your genetic makeup is like an architectural blueprint for a building. We each have our own unique blueprint that dictates how our house (our body) gets built. And although the specifications are fairly scripted, how those specifications are interpreted and acted upon will determine the long-term resilience and longevity of the structure.

The three little pigs all had the same blueprint instruction: Build a house. But each pig chose different raw materials with very different results. If you build your home with inferior materials, you will have more maintenance problems and the home will not last as long as it would have had you used superior materials and careful craftsmanship. Likewise for the same genetic code (identical twins, for example) — health outcomes can be very different, depending on individual lifestyle choices.

Sometimes, building plans can result in a really sturdy structure even when the building materials are of lesser quality. There's always a story around about the uncle who lived to be "a hundred" even though he ate only potato chips and chain smoked unfiltered cigarettes. OK — cool. But can you imagine how long (and well) he might have lived if he had eaten a balanced diet and respected his lungs? Just because he lucked into an awesome architectural plan (good genes) doesn't mean he maximized the full benefit of the plans. No doubt genetics can help you. Just please don't squander your natural advantage.

> *Regardless of the blueprint you bring to the table, build with bricks, not with straw!*

Certain families seem to have really bad blueprints. The building plans their bodies follow appear to be flawed, resulting in especially flimsy structures constructed over and over again. These are the families with histories of heart disease or strokes in younger family members, often with multiple relatives involved. A lot of attention and vigilance is absolutely essential in such situations.

Blood is thicker

It is imperative that you take the time to find out as much as you can about the health of your relatives — your blood relatives. Your spouse and their relatives, or your step-relatives and their families, are not material to this discussion.

From a heart perspective, you are interested in finding out whether anyone in your family (your brothers, sisters, parents, cousins, aunts, uncles, and grandparents) ever had a heart attack, stroke, angioplasty, bypass surgery, or aneurysm. If any of those relatives have passed away, you should try to find out approximately how old they were when they died and the cause of death.

You're history

The U.S. Department of Health and Human Services (HHS) Family History Initiative has an excellent Web site at (www.hhs.gov/familyhistory). It has a tool called "My Family History Portrait," which allows you to compile, save, and update a family history of health problems. This site suggests you update the family history regularly — like at events where family members gather, such as Thanksgiving. In fact, the Surgeon General declared Thanksgiving 2005 a National Family History Day.

As long as you're asking all these questions, you should also ask about cancers — especially breast and colon cancer — as well as about diabetes, osteoporosis, and Alzheimer's disease. The more you know about the health histories of your relatives, the better picture you'll get of your own blueprint and the sort of structure you are inclined to build.

Ask one or two people to take on the task of compiling the family health history and pass that on to the other family members. This can be a daunting task, especially since these days family members are more likely to live far from each other and may see each other only occasionally. But the effort to compile these data is well worth it. The data can contain major clues about what you need to watch out for. And, as if watching out for your own health wasn't benefit enough, remember that your family's genetic history can very well affect your children.

Family history

OK, what if your family includes one or more relatives who have had heart disease? Step one: Don't panic. Step two: Get more curious. Step three: Take action!

If the relatives with heart disease were younger (especially male relatives with heart disease before the age of 55 and female relatives with heart disease before the age of 65) or if multiple relatives developed heart disease regardless of their ages, you really need to get more information — about your relatives and about yourself.

Try to obtain information about the risk factors of your relatives with the heart disease. Were they diabetic? Did they smoke? Did they have high blood pressure or high cholesterol? And was the diagnosis of heart disease actually confirmed or was it presumed?

For yourself, find out your prevention status and what you can do to improve your chances, that is, what you can do to build a better building despite the flawed plans you were handed. This is where knowing your numbers is imperative and keeping yourself (and your physician) on task to optimize all those numbers becomes incredibly important. I'm not implying that if you don't have a family history you get to be a slacker about prevention efforts. But if anyone needs to be almost obsessed with this stuff, it's the person with a strong family history of heart disease.

The person with a family history of heart disease is also the person who often needs to go the extra mile in detecting risk factors and quantifying their plaque buildup. Patients with a significant family history of heart disease often benefit from advanced blood testing (lipoprotein A, C-reactive protein, homocysteine, LDL and HDL sub fractions, and the like), and occasionally from CT scans or other imaging of their heart or blood vessels. They also should be extra vigilant about their cholesterol levels, aiming for an LDL cholesterol goal one category lower than would be advised if they didn't have a strong family history. If you've forgotten what those goals should be, go back and review those chapters again. *This is really important!* If you have a significant family history of heart disease and you are not following all the advice in this book, you are playing with fire. You are building a house of straw, and it won't take a lot of huffing or puffing to blow you down.

Piece of Advice #15

Talk to your relatives about your family's health history. You want to specifically hone in on the occurrence of heart disease, stroke, aneurysm, cancer, hypertension, and diabetes. Write down that information and organize it by mother's side and father's side and by generation. Share the information (and the information-gathering process if feasible) with your siblings and your children. Make a copy of your findings for your physician.

*Visit **www.CardioSmart.org** for tools to help you calculate your risk for heart disease*

CHAPTER 18

To Stress a Point...

If you ask me what is the single most important key to
longevity, I would have to say it is avoiding worry, stress
and tension. And if you didn't ask me, I'd still have to say it.
— GEORGE BURNS (1896–1996)

A while ago, I read a very good book about diabetes care aimed at patients with this disease, *Understand Your Diabetes and Live a Healthy Life*. The book included a chapter about stress and stress management and presented this topic in a very understandable format while providing sound advice. If you are a diabetic, I would encourage you to read this book for an excellent overview of diabetes and how you can affect your blood sugars and overall care. I have borrowed from this book the themes presented about stress and have adapted them for the purposes of our discussion. It turns out you don't have to be diabetic to be negatively affected by stress. We are all potentially at risk for the negative effects of this life force. Read on ...

Are you a serious person? Brooding? Anxious? Do you find that your life is very stressful? It turns out that those emotions aren't just unpleasant to experience, they are also potentially harmful to our bodies.

Research into stress and depression, as well as into aggressive personality traits, has shown that the way we handle stress and the stress we are exposed to contributes to heart disease, aging, cancer, and immune dysfunction.

Fight or flight

Stress. You can't avoid it. It is an inescapable part of our lives. And it is not necessarily bad. But recurrent stress, chronic stress, or stress that affects our ability to function at our best can be harmful over the long haul.

I'm often asked if stress *causes* heart disease. The short answer: It's complicated. Stress in and of itself is not the issue. But the body's response to that stress can be devastating, especially in the appropriately predisposed individual.

While under stress, the body is in a state of "fight or flight" — an adaptive mechanism whereby the body is geared to either engage the "enemy" in battle (e.g., face the demanding boss) or escape the threat as fast as possible (e.g., use the back hall to get to the lunch room and thereby avoid her office). In either circumstance, all systems must be in the "go" position. The body needs to have a lot of readily available energy to act and be hormonally triggered toward aggression and maximal vigilance against the looming threat.

So what? Well, glucose is the fastest and easiest energy source we can access, so stress can increase blood sugar levels. Increased glucose causes insulin release. (Sugar and insulin; they just keep coming up over and over and over again!) Remember, insulin is a storage hormone that pushes cholesterol pathways toward favoring formation of LDL. Adrenaline, one of the hormones released in response to stress, lowers our tissues' sensitivity toward insulin, thereby driving blood sugars (and LDL) higher. Adrenaline also increases blood pressure levels.

It is not hard to see that stress can push people having a predisposition toward high blood sugars, high LDL, or hypertension over the edge. Furthermore, because stress is a distraction, risk-factor control might worsen simply because we are preoccupied — not paying attention to our food intake or our exercise schedule. We might also reach for comforting things like ice cream and candy bars, or increase or resume our tobacco habit.

Heartbreaker

If that's not enough, an acute or sudden change in stress level can cause very rapid changes in physiology. The sudden blood pressure rise or the sudden change in blood biochemistry can be just enough to trigger a sudden disruption of vulnerable endothelium, leading to a heart attack or stroke.

In cases of sudden extreme stress, some people literally develop a "broken heart." The very high levels of stress hormones released stun the heart muscle, causing the heart to pump blood very poorly. This sudden change can cause such reduced blood supply to the liver, kidneys, and brain that these organs begin to fail and individuals may require transient life support therapy. This series of events is not due to coronary artery disease — indeed these individuals actually have normal coronary arteries. This is purely due to acute stress hormone overload. This is a very rare complication of extreme stress, but underscores the connection between the heart and the brain.

Now don't start thinking that every time you're under stress you're a ticking time bomb or that you require immediate medical attention. From a heart perspective, your individual vulnerability toward the negative effects of stress is directly proportional to your individual vulnerability of developing heart disease in general. Smokers or people with blood sugar abnormalities, blood pressure issues, excess weight, or high LDL will be at higher risk from stress than individuals without such health issues.

Taking steps to prevent heart disease means you take steps to ward off the negative and potentially life-threatening effects of stress.

What is stress? A good definition would be the feeling *you* get when *you* perceive a situation as threatening and feel as though *you* can't deal well with that situation.

You is emphasized in the definition because stress is extremely person specific. Stress depends on one's perception of the situation at hand — and that perception can vary extremely from person to person and from situation to situation.

Stress can be a positive force. A challenging situation can be stimulating and finding the solution rewarding, resulting in tremendous personal satisfaction and increased self-esteem. Only when the stress is the result of feeling unable to deal with a situation does it become a negative force and result in the myriad physiologic responses described above.

The visual example of stress beyond control that I keep in the back of my mind is a movie about a classic rat experiment I saw during my Psychology 101 class many (*many*) years ago. If you've ever studied psychology, I'm sure you are familiar with this experiment. It's an excellent example of the effects of stress over time. The basic construct consisted of a rat working through a maze or doing different activities in some box. Regardless of the path the rat chose in the maze or the activity it attempted, it would receive a painful shock.

Initially, the rat would try to figure out ways to prevent getting shocked — it would appear hyperaware and engaged with its surroundings. As the experiment continued and the rat continued to receive shocks regardless of what it did, it became progressively less active, and eventually retreated to a corner where it cowered and trembled. The rat was so stressed by its surroundings and situation that it was no longer able to function. What started out as an adaptation (hyperawareness, excitement to outsmart the shocks), progressed to a maladaptive response — an almost opposite reaction of withdrawal and submission. Keep the rat in mind as you read about how people respond to stress and how those responses manifest themselves in different ways.

Stress deconstructed

All enemies are more easily defeated one unit at a time. The same is true of stress, as examined in these units —

- **Sources of stress.** People find many sources of stress, many different sources of those electric shocks. Major, unpleasant life changes such as a divorce or illness are readily recognized as stressful. But even happy events (such as marriages, the birth of a child, or career advancements) may be equally stressful. *The common denominator is change — change can be very stressful.*

- **Response to stress.** The way we respond to the stress determines the effect that stress has on our bodies. An individual's personality, previous experiences, and ability to adapt will have a huge impact on the way they handle stress initially (each rat brings different baggage to the cage). Luckily (or sometimes not so luckily), we are not alone in the cage and our support network, or people or circumstances adding to our burdens, may affect the degree and duration of the stress.

- **Symptoms of stress.** What are the symptoms of stress? They fall into three broad categories: Physical symptoms, emotional symptoms, and behavioral changes. The physical signs that may indicate that you are under stress include a rapid heartbeat, increased blood pressure readings, and faster breathing rate. Remember, you are getting ready for fight or flight! These physical changes could be considered generally adaptive to the situation, but that does not mean that these changes are necessarily beneficial — especially if they are long-lasting due to ongoing stress, and especially if you are at increased risk for developing heart disease or its complications.

Some physical symptoms of adrenaline overdrive (where the physical stress response is maladaptive: You're feeling like you're getting shocked no matter what you do; you're cowering in the corner of the cage) may include headaches, digestive problems, fatigue, muscle tension, and even chest tightness or pain.

I have seen many patients who present with symptoms of chest pain similar to that of angina, which, after thorough investigation, turn out to be related to unresolved stress rather than significant underlying coronary artery disease. These patients weren't crazy or imagining their pain, and their pain wasn't in their heads. Their symptoms were very real and for some, very frightening. Their chest pains were their bodies' ways of signaling that they were on stress overdrive and in need of stress relief. They were trembling in the corner of their cages.

I tell you this *not* to have you ignore any symptoms you may have and attribute them to stress. *If you have symptoms that may be related to heart disease — for heaven's sake, see your doctor!* Stress can be assumed the cause of symptoms only once potentially serious alternate explanations have been ruled out. So if you experience chest discomfort, unusual shortness of breath or exercise intolerance, regardless of your stress levels, don't ignore these symptoms! Discuss them with your doctor.

- **Other signs of stress.** Emotional/behavioral signs of stress may include not only aggression (as expected, and relatively adaptive), but also (with stress overdrive) depression, reduced concentration/motivation, and even loss of self-esteem (visualize that rat!). People who are under stress, especially chronic stress, may feel empty, dissatisfied, or even ambivalent about their situations. People under stress are frequently irritable, and tend toward arguing easily. They may become forgetful and display a reduction in productivity. Sexual drive may decline. Use of tobacco, alcohol and other addictive substances may increase. Food consumption often becomes less mindful and calorie ingestion may increase substantially — especially in those individuals who identify themselves as emotional eaters.

Uncaged

Experiencing stress is no day at the beach and its presence can wreak havoc with our bodies and our emotions. This is why it is so important to balance and control the stress in our lives. We have to get out of that cage!

How do we get out?

Well, the first step is recognizing that each of us is in a cage. This can actually be quite challenging — the recognition that you have a problem — especially if you are in stress overdrive. You have to be able to understand your sources of stress and your level of stress. Are you hyperaware and engaged (good) or are you withdrawing, angry or depressed (bad)? Are you able to devote time and attention to your health and personal relationships (good) or are you ignoring your body and your health by being continually preoccupied with external demands (bad)?

You need to identify which stresses are positive forces for you and which are not. Maybe the job promotion is just the thing you need to keep you interested in your work. But maybe the dread of more responsibilities and increased time pressures has your stomach in knots. Be honest with yourself about your feelings and responses. There are no right or wrong answers here — this is all about what works and doesn't work *for you.*

Deal with it

Next, you have to come up with some ways to deal with your unwanted stress. The plan should look something like this:

- Define the problem or stress provoker.

- Come up with as many solutions to improve the situation as you can.

- Decide which approach is easiest to implement and most likely to succeed.

- Commit to the solution, and make the changes you need to make.

Yeah, right! This sounds so concrete and logical and our problems are so complex and messy. But you have to create order from chaos if your existence is going to change. And you don't necessarily have to do this alone. Many trained professionals — from counselors and social workers to psychologists and psychiatrists — can help. And you probably have a support network already, whether it's made up of family, friends, co-workers or spiritual leaders. It's OK to ask for help or guidance. Sometimes we can only get out of the cage if someone helps pull us out.

Positively healthy

My main goal for including this chapter has been to point out that *our emotional lives and our reactions to the events around us affect our health and, consequently, our longevity.* You respond to your surroundings not only emotionally, but also very physically. Although a person can't always control his or her environment, the way he or she chooses to react to that environment influences not just that person's sense of happiness, but also his or her heart's health.

I've spent time talking mostly about stress and maladaptive responses. But remember, just as negative emotions can have a negative impact, positive emotions can have a positive impact.

Life truly is short! We only go around once! Yes, the ride can be bumpy, but isn't life fantastic anyway? Please don't waste precious time by relentlessly fretting over what might happen or what might have been. Try to live with positive emotions!

Breathe. Relax. Do something just for yourself. Try to fulfill some of your dreams and nurture your talents. Contribute to causes you believe in — no, not just monetarily, but with action. Rekindle old friendships and make new friends. Reconnect with your family. Opening your heart to others is one of the keys to finding purpose and a connection to the world.

Add laughter to your life and take yourself less seriously. Try to see the glass as half full. Marvel at the miracles all around you — your children; the earth, sky, and stars; your beating heart. Be grateful for all your blessings. Take time to pray. Hug the people you love. Laugh. Every day.

Piece of Advice #16

Make the preceding paragraph an everyday action list for yourself. If you need to, photocopy the list and review it daily.

Take myself less seriously.
Try to see the glass as half full.
Marvel at the miracles all around me.
Be grateful for all my blessings.
Hug the people I love.
Take time to pray.
Laugh.
Every day.

And if despite all your efforts, you still have a tough time dealing with stress, or feel blue or anxious much of the time, or really can't find joy in your life, please take the time to talk with your doctor.

CHAPTER 19

I Am Woman, Hear Me Roar

Women who seek to be equal with men lack ambition.
— TIMOTHY LEARY (1920–1996)

Heart disease is the number one killer and disabler of women in this country. It takes the lives of more women than all cancer deaths *combined*. And that includes breast cancer.

And although the message is getting out there, many women continue to ignore their risks, and more importantly, ignore their symptoms..

So far, it appears men and women share risk factors. The proportional effect of a particular risk may vary between the sexes (we are still investigating this), but for all intents and purposes, everything I have written about in this book applies to both men and women.

But ...

Women are different

Women and men differ in many important ways. In general, women are smaller (not necessarily lighter — I'm talking about lean body mass here). And being smaller means that they have smaller organs and smaller coronary arteries. So a smaller amount of plaque can gum up their systems. A smaller clot can obstruct downstream flow and result in a heart attack. And because the arteries are smaller to begin with, they're more technically challenging to bypass and to stent, so that the procedural results in women are not always as good and not always as long lasting as they are in men.

Scientists have recently observed that the way atherosclerosis builds up in women might be different as compared to men. Women can develop **small vessel disease**; that is, instead of blockages affecting the three main coronary arteries, blockages primarily affect the branches of those arteries — branches that are too small for us to see very well with an angiogram or to treat with bypass surgery or angioplasty.

So women have a smaller reserve to begin with and less wiggle room for therapy if it's needed. Which is maybe why 38 percent of women who have a heart attack will die within one year. We have to stop being statistics!

Lady's a man

Women are blessed (?) with a very distinct hormonal milieu for a good chunk of their lives. And that hormonal milieu appears to be protective. There's something about the estrogen floating around in our bloodstreams that seems to ward off heart disease, at least temporarily. This is probably nature's way of ensuring we will be around long enough to raise our children. But as kids go off to college and we hit menopause, all hell breaks loose. In fact, following menopause (natural or surgical), within a very short period of time, we catch up to men and their relative heart disease risk. So ladies, from a heart disease perspective, about 10 years after your last period, you're a man.

We have already touched on the issue of hormonal supplementation earlier in this book. For emphasis, current data do not support use of hormone supplements as an effective means of reducing heart disease risk in women. In fact, several trials have pointed to a higher risk of heart attacks in women taking hormone supplements. As with all studies, however, the results obtained in a controlled group of specifically selected subjects may not translate well to every woman in the real world. Hormone supplementation can still be considered for treatment of menopausal symptoms, but in general, using the lowest effective dose for the shortest amount of time probably makes sense. As with all things in medicine, hormone supplementation remains an evolving story. If you currently take hormone supplements or are contemplating starting, discuss the anticipated duration of therapy, the various types of supplements and dosage options with your physician. And don't rely on hormone supplements for the prevention of heart disease. Instead, concentrate on optimizing your weight, eating plan, exercise regimen, cholesterol profile, blood pressure readings, and blood sugar levels. And for goodness sake, stop smoking!

Ellen's diabetes

Women with diabetes appear to be an especially high-risk group not only for developing heart disease, but also for faring worse with any available treatment for heart disease. Diabetes actually wipes out estrogen's protective effect so even young women of childbearing age who have diabetes have a very high risk of developing heart disease. (Remember Ellen, the patient behind this book.)

If there's one kind of patient I worry about (a lot), it's the woman with diabetes. If you are a woman with diabetes (regardless of your need for insulin), *please* be extra vigilant about your risks and your symptoms. The earlier you get your other risk factors under control and the earlier you seek treatment for your symptoms, the better chance you will have of living a long and healthy life. If your diabetes is partially or largely due to excess weight, make every effort humanly possible to lose that weight and lose that diabetes. Your risk outlook will change dramatically.

When compared to men, women seem to have different symptoms when they present with heart disease — perhaps this explains why women until recently have been largely ignored in terms of testing and treatment. The classic description of **angina** (a squeezing or heavy sensation experienced diffusely over the chest, radiating down the arm and up into the neck) is a description much more likely to be given by a man than a woman. Although a woman can experience such symptoms, she can also present with weakness or fatigue, shortness of breath, a burning sensation in the chest more like heartburn or indigestion, or an atypical discomfort located in the jaw, shoulder, neck, back or a localized chest area.

Heartburn, pain and fatigue!

OK, I probably have you spooked right now. If you're a woman reading this chapter, you're probably thinking — hey, I've had heartburn and pain in my shoulder. Yesterday I was winded climbing the steps. And fatigue? — tell me about it!! Well, even if you have had any one or more of these symptoms you don't necessarily have heart disease. We still have to put those symptoms into context by looking at your risk factor profile and your age. If you are high risk (because you are a 70-year-old hypertensive smoker, or because you are a diabetic of any age), we need to look further into these symptoms. If you are a young woman without any risk factors, your presentations is still unlikely to be indicative of coronary disease, even if "classic."

The point I'm making is this: *We need to throw out the notion that a woman presenting with atypical symptoms can't have heart disease — especially if she has risk factors, and especially if she's a woman with diabetes.*

Women have a unique role in society. We are caretakers — of our children, of our spouses, of our parents, of our friends. We also need to be caretakers of our hearts. The heart disease statistics for our gender are appalling. By becoming more proactive in our care and more involved in prevention efforts, we can change those statistics, ensuring that we'll not only see our children go off to college, but we'll also see our grandchildren graduate from college.

And as we take better care of ourselves, we'll take better care of those we love. Not just because we'll be around longer, but because we can influence the health habits of our children, our spouses and even our parents (sometimes, on a good day, if they'd just listen!).

Piece of Advice #17

If you are a woman and have never discussed heart disease prevention with your physician, make an appointment and get started. Many of us see only our gynecologists with any regularity and might not have any other health-care providers. Not all gynecologists are well versed in cardiovascular prevention guidelines and therapies. It's OK to ask your provider if he or she is comfortable advising you. If he or she is not, ask for a referral to a physician who can take on that role. This is important. Take action!

CHAPTER 20

Putting It *All* Together

A goal without a plan is just a wish.
— Antoine de Saint-Exupery (1900–1944)

Here's a recap of this book's major points. Sometimes it's nice to see a quick reference to jog your memory and nudge you into action.

Heart disease:

- Heart disease is the number one killer and disabler in our country, claiming a life every 35 seconds.
- Heart disease is predominantly preventable and can be avoided with strict control of all modifiable risk factors.
- Heart disease is a stealthy disease and may progress inside your body without your detecting any symptoms.
- Heart disease may make itself known with a sudden, major, life-altering event *out of the blue* if you ignore any risk factors you may have.

Stress tests:

- A normal stress test, though reassuring and a good baseline, does not mean that you don't have any coronary artery disease.
- A normal stress test result is *not* a free pass to making poor lifestyle choices or to ignoring *any* risk factors you may have for developing heart disease.

Risk factors:

- The same risk factors that cause gunk to build up inside our arteries also make the endothelium more vulnerable to breaking down and make plaque unstable. Here's that list:

  — Smoking
  — High blood pressure
  — Cholesterol abnormalities
  — Diabetes
  — Inactivity
  — Poor diet
  — Excess weight
  — A family history of heart disease
  — Increasing age

- Controlling your risk factors not only prevents the need for bypass surgery and stents but also prevents the occurrence of heart attacks.

Cholesterol:

- A **standard cholesterol profile** contains the total cholesterol and the three main particles that make up that total: HDL, LDL and triglycerides.
- The **total cholesterol number** is the least useful statistic from this whole profile, so if you want one less thing to remember, forget the total cholesterol.

- Knowing your **HDL, LDL and TG levels** on the other hand is vital to being an active and informed participant in your personal crusade to ward off heart disease.
- **HDL** particles can be thought of as garbage trucks. These cholesterol particles do not deposit cholesterol in your arteries — they are removing cholesterol from your body. You want this number as high as possible. In general, levels below 40 are worrisome and levels above 60 are encouraging.
- **LDL** can be thought of as bags of garbage, and the cholesterol that deposits in your arteries. You want this number to be as low as possible — by my estimate definitely below 130 mg/dL, ideally below 100 mg/dL, and in certain circumstances below 70 mg/dL.
- The **total cholesterol to HDL ratio** can be helpful in sorting out situations where the HDL and LDL levels provide conflicting signals regarding your risk. This ratio should be below 4.
- **Triglycerides** (TG) are a health risk when very high on their own (especially >1000 mg/dL) because of the increased risk of pancreatitis. Triglyceride elevation as an isolated finding contributes to heart disease risk but probably not as powerfully as abnormalities of HDL or LDL levels. Normal TG levels are defined as less than 150 mg/dL.
- The combination of low HDL and high triglycerides is a particularly toxic one and is referred to as **metabolic syndrome**. Patients with metabolic syndrome are at an especially high risk for developing heart disease over time. This type of profile requires a rapid and concerted effort to normalize the numbers.
- All **cholesterol abnormalities** tend to improve with healthful lifestyle changes. Triglycerides are most sensitive to lifestyle changes while HDL is least sensitive. Regardless of the magnitude of change however, a healthful diet, regular exercise and attainment and maintenance of a sensible weight are basic cornerstones of cholesterol management.
- For adults, it is reasonable to start **measuring your cholesterol profile** in your 20s, at the very least by 30 years of age, unless marked cholesterol abnormalities occur in close relatives, you have a very early family history of heart disease, or you are diabetic — in which case starting the measurements earlier is

appropriate. The frequency of subsequent measurements depends upon the findings, and your overall health status. Discuss your particular situation with your doctor to come up with a reasonable monitoring plan.

Additional testing:

- **Markers of heart disease risk** above and beyond a cholesterol profile may reveal additional information about your particular situation.
- These markers can be measured with **blood tests**, although some require specialized laboratories to perform the analyses and the tests may be expensive. All of these additional tests should be considered for patients with personal or family histories of early or accelerated heart disease.

  — Everyone should have their **lipoprotein A level** checked at least once in their lives.
  — **LDL and HDL sub fraction analysis** should probably be reserved for those situations in which, despite other testing, the reason for an accelerated atherosclerotic process is unclear.
  — Patients with accelerated atherosclerosis or a strong family history of CAD should probably have their **homocysteine level** evaluated.
  — The story about **C-reactive protein** is still evolving. This test may become more widely used for risk assessment as more data emerges. At the present time, using this test as a double check on the completeness of prevention efforts seems reasonable.

- In general, if an **abnormality** of any of these additional markers exists, it is a signal that your prevention efforts need to kick into higher gear — from crossing all the *t*'s and dotting all the *i*'s in your diet, exercise program, and weight control efforts to tightening the goals for components of the regular cholesterol profile.

Blood pressure:

- **Hypertension** is a major contributor to heart disease, and the number one preventable cause of heart failure.
- A **normal blood pressure** is defined as less than or equal to 120/80 mmHg. Both the systolic and diastolic numbers are important, although the systolic (top number) reading is often used for assessment of blood pressure control. You should be concerned if you are seeing blood pressure readings over 130 mmHg systolic or 85 mmHg diastolic at your health checkups. Readings persistently over 140/90 mmHg require blood pressure lowering medications.
- Obesity, tobacco use, lack of exercise, high sodium consumption, and sleep apnea are all **contributors to hypertension** that can be modified or reversed. Control what you have control over.
- If your readings are not optimal, become an active participant in your care by becoming more involved in **monitoring of your blood pressure readings**. A home monitor is relatively inexpensive and can be extremely effective and helpful in guiding your care. Know your readings and where you fall on the spectrum of blood pressure categories. Do not accept advice to watch abnormal readings unless you have a clear plan about what action to take regarding those readings. Hypertension is a modifiable risk factor. Watching your blood pressure does nothing to modify your risk.
- Many **medications** lower blood pressure. An effective program can be devised for your particular situation. Please be patient with your health-care provider. At times it requires several attempts at different dosages or combinations of medications to attain the desired result. The important part is to establish a goal and, within a reasonable time, to attain that goal.
- **Your actions** contribute to your blood pressure. How you live your life, how you control your weight and what you eat can have a dramatic effect on your blood pressure control. Be proactive in your own care.

Smoking:

- If you **smoke**, you must quit!

Blood sugar and diabetes:

- Abnormally **elevated blood sugar levels** are common, affecting approximately *one in five* Americans.

  — **Chronically elevated glucose levels** lead to blood vessel, nerve and organ damage. The number one cause of death in diabetics is cardiovascular disease.
  — An **abnormal fasting glucose level** is defined as any number above 100 mg/dL. Recurring values above 125 mg/dL define the presence of full-blown diabetes.
  — Even intermediate **fasting blood glucose (FBG)** levels (those between 100 and 125 mg/dL) are very worrisome and require an all-out effort to reverse this abnormality.
  — The vast majority of diabetics have **type 2 diabetes**, which is closely linked to excess weight and lack of physical activity.

- If your sugars are elevated, work with your physician and your health-care team to bring those values down ASAP.

- **Move your body** and, if you're overweight, **lose those excess pounds** — this is your best chance to eliminate your sugar woes and reduce your long-term health risks.

Weight:

- **Obesity and excess weight** are extremely common in our society and associated with a multitude of health risks and a shortened life span.

  — To assess your own status, use the **BMI table** (chapter 14) to determine your body mass index. Anything over 25 is concerning. Anything over 30 is a *weight emergency.*

— Your waist measurement is another clue to impending disaster — if it's 40 inches or more in a man or 35 inches or more in a woman, it's a call to action.

- There are no magic solutions to excess weight — it's calories in versus calories out. If you take in more than you expend, you will gain weight. The only way to lose weight is to eat less and move more.

Food:

- Choose your foods wisely. **Garbage in equals garbage out.** Don't be a trash can.
- Consume food in reasonable quantities. **Portion control** is weight control.
- Enjoy a wide **variety of foods** from every food category. Deprivation does not work. But this does not cancel out the garbage rule — junk is junk is junk and you should not eat it.
- Increase your intake of **fruits and vegetables**. Raw! Raw! Raw!
- Add **beans and legumes** to your diet as a substitute for meat and to add fiber.
- Choose **water and tea** as beverages. Dilute all fruit juices with water.
- Start **preparing more of your food**. Control is power.
- Stop **snacking**.
- Balance any obvious **dietary indiscretions**.
- And always remember to **savor and enjoy** your food — stop fighting with it!

Exercise:

- It's a **vital component of a healthy existence** that needs to be as much a part of your day as is brushing your teeth or eating a meal.
- **Thirty minutes** of daily exercise is the *minimum*. We should

be aiming to move our bodies for 60 to 90 minutes per day. If the minimum is too much right now, do what you can. It *all counts.*

- **Longer periods** of exercise are more beneficial at building endurance and more likely to improve your fitness level.
- If you can't devote longer periods during the day, incorporating 30 to 90 minutes of **movement divided into small chunks** is still beneficial because of the increased calorie expenditure.
- Enjoy a **mix of activities** that allow for both aerobic training and muscle building. Avoid muscle building exclusively as a workout regimen.
- **Weight management** is all about calories in versus calories out. Burn baby burn!

Family history:

- Find out as much as you can about the **health history** of your blood relatives.
- **Early development of heart disease** in your relatives or the finding of multiple relatives with heart disease should cause you to kick your own prevention efforts into high gear.

Stress:

- It can have a **negative impact on heart disease risk**, especially in those patients with poorly controlled risk factors to begin with.
- **Chronic stress** can lead to increased blood pressures, increased blood sugar, and loss of focus in maintaining a healthy nutrient intake and exercise routine.
- A major component of dealing with bad stress is **recognizing that stress is present** and that it affects you negatively.
- **Seek help** if you are having difficulties coping, are angry or negative much of the time, or have lost interest or pleasure in your daily activities.

Women's concerns:

- **Heart disease kills more women** than all cancer deaths *combined*.
- The same **risk factors** that are important to men are also significant to women, although relative impact may be different for any given risk factor.
- **Hormone replacement therapy** is probably not very effective in reducing the risk of heart disease. Women are better off controlling all "traditional" risk factors, rather than relying on hormone replacement for heart health maintenance.
- Women may present with **unusual or atypical symptoms**. Those symptoms should not be ignored, especially in women with significant risk factors for heart disease or women with diabetes.
- **Diabetes** wipes out any natural advantage that women have in delaying the process of plaque buildup. Diabetic women are an especially high-risk group for the development of heart disease and for experiencing complications from heart disease.
- Women need to become more proactive in their **risk factor management** and need to seek out physicians interested and knowledgeable in this endeavor.

·

And finally, we return to the beginning. Here's that original list of pledges to live by every single day:

> *I will take back control of my life and make it better.*

> *I will stop putting junk in my mouth because I know that garbage in means garbage out.*

> *I will move my body every day.*

> *I will stop all harmful behaviors that are under my control.*

> *I will learn about heart disease and maintenance of heart health — because knowledge is power.*

> *I will acquire a good understanding of all my personal risk factors for heart disease and work hard to neutralize them as much as I can.*

> *I will do all of this because if I don't, I will die.*

Conclusion
and Reality Check

The big secret in life
is that there is no big secret.
Whatever your goal, you can
get there if you're willing to work.
— Oprah Winfrey

I hope you are inspired by some of the things you have read in this book. My whole goal is to get as many people as I can interested in preventing heart disease and doing something about it.

However, I would be lying if I said that I, myself, follow every piece of advice in this book 100 percent of the time. There were times when I was writing this book just as much for myself and my family as for you and yours. I struggle all the time with providing nutritious meals for my family and finding time to exercise. My husband struggles with losing weight and keeping it off. This stay-healthy stuff can be really hard! I never said that slaying the giant would be easy. But we don't have the option of giving up just because it's a struggle. The stakes are simply too high.

None of us is perfect. And it's so much easier *not* to follow the advice in this book. But every positive change you make is a positive change for your heart and your health. You don't have to make them all at once: Examine what you can do better, what pieces of information you are missing about your health, and commit to doing your absolute best to minimize your risk for developing heart disease over time. Make a commitment to your heart and your health every single day. Your life really does depend upon it.

This is it. You won't ever get a chance to repeat today. *Every* action is important. *Every* action has an effect. *Everything* is cumulative. *Every* bad choice affects your health over time. And every *good* choice brings you one step forward on the road to a long and vital existence.

You can do it! You can slay the giant! And know that every step of the way I'll be out there cheering you on.

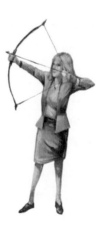

Appendix: Metric Measurements

HDL Basics in Metric (mmol/L)

Optimal HDL level:

Over 1.37 for men; over 1.74 for premenopausal women (this is often averaged to 1.55 for everyone; bottom line—the higher the better!)

Acceptable HDL level:

Over 1.04 for men and postmenopausal women; over 1.30 for premenopausal women

Get help!

Under 0.96 for men and postmenopausal women, under 1.22 for premenopausal women (this is often averaged to 1.04 for everyone; bottom line—the higher the better!)

LDL Basics in Metric (mmol/L)

Current published recommendations: (at the very least your numbers should reflect these)	
Minimum goal for everyone	below 4.14
Minimum goal if you have any risk factors	below 3.37
Minimum goal if you have coronary disease or coronary disease equivalent	below 2.59
Get help!	over 4.14

More aggressive goals: (the goals more and more cardiologists recommend)	
Minimum goal for everyone	below 3.37
Minimum goal if you have any risk factors	below 2.59
Minimum goal if you have coronary disease or coronary disease equivalent	below 1.81
Get help!	over 3.37

Triglyceride Basics in Metric (mmol/L)

Current published recommendations:	
Ideal for everyone	below 1.70
Worry about metabolic syndrome	over 1.70
Get help!	over 4.52

Lipoprotein A in Metric (mmol/L)

Ideally below 0.78

Homocysteine in Metric (umol/L)

Ideally below 2.03

Blood Sugar Basics in Metric (mmol/L)

Normal	below 5.55
Pre-diabetes	5.56 to 6.94
Diabetes	6.95 or higher

References

Abraham WT. 2005. New approaches in the prevention of heart failure. *Textbook of Cardiovascular Medicine Updates.* 8(4):1–12.

American Heart Association. *Heart Disease and Stroke Statistics — 2005 Update.* http://www.americanheart.org/downloadable/heart/1105390918119HDSStats2005Update.pdf

American Heart Association. *Statistical Fact Sheet: Populations. Women and Cardiovascular Diseases: Statistics.* http://www.americanheart.org/downloadable/heart/1104938287787FS10WM05rev.pdf

Appel LJ et al. 2005. Effect of protein, monounsaturated fat and carbohydrate intake on blood pressure and serum lipids. Results of the OmniHeart Randomized Trial. *JAMA*, 294:2455–2464.

Ballantyne CM et al. 2005. Lipoprotein-associated phospholipase A2, high sensitivity C-Reactive protein, and risk for incident ischemic stroke in middle-aged men and women in the Atherosclerosis Risk in Communities (ARIC) study. *Arch Intern Med*, 165:2479–2484.

Berger JS et al. 2006. Aspirin for the primary prevention of cardiovascular events in women and men: A sex-specific meta-analysis of randomized controlled trials. *JAMA*, 295:306–313.

Bhatt DL et al. 2006. International prevalence, recognition, and treatment of cardiovascular risk factors in outpatients with atherothrombosis. *JAMA*, 295:180–189.

Blackburn GL & Waltman BA. 2005. Physician's guide to the new 2005 dietary guidelines: How best to counsel patients. *Clev Clin J Med*, 72:609–618.

Broeder C et al. 1992. The effects of either high intensity resistance or endurance training on resting metabolic rate. *Am J Clin Nutr*, 55:802–810.

Brown AS, ed. 2005. A symposium: Impending epidemic of obesity, metabolic syndrome and diabetes mellitus — the role of prevention. *Am J Card*, 96(Suppl 4A):1E–69E.

Brown L et al. 1999. Cholesterol-lowering effects of dietary fiber: A meta-analysis. *Am J Clin Nutr,* 69:30–42.

Cannon CP et al. 2004 Intensive versus moderate lipid lowering with statins after acute coronary syndromes. *N Engl J Med,* 350:1495–1504.

Chobanian AV et al. 2003. Seventh report of the Joint National Committee on Prevention, Detection, Evaluation, and Treatment of High Blood Pressure. *Hypertension,* 42:1206–1252.

Cholesterol Treatment Trialists' (CCT) Collaborators. 2005. Efficacy and safety of cholesterol lowering treatment: Prospective meta-analysis of data from 90,056 participants in 14 randomised trials of statins. *Lancet,* 366:1267–1278.

Christen WG et al. 2000. Blood levels of homocysteine and increased risks of cardiovascular disease: Causal or casual? *Arch Intern Med,* 160:422–434.

Citkowitz E. *Hypertriglyceridemia.* http://www.emedicine.com/med/topic2921.htm

Colohoun HM et al. 2004. Primary prevention of cardiovascular disease with atorvastatin in type 2 diabetes in the Collaborative Atorvastatin Diabetes Study (CARDS): Multicenter randomized placebo-controlled trial. *Lancet,* 364:685–696.

Cui Y et al. 2001. Non-high-density lipoprotein cholesterol level as a predictor of cardiovascular disease mortality. *Arch Intern Med,* 161:1413–1419.

Cushman M et al. 2005. C-reactive protein and the 10-year incidence of coronary heart disease in older men and women: The Cardiovascular Health Study. *Circulation,* 112:25–31.

Dansinger ML et al. 2005. Comparison of the Atkins, Ornish, Weight Watchers, and Zone diets for weight loss and heart disease risk reduction — A randomized trial. *JAMA,* 293:43–53.

Diabetes Day Care Unit, Understand Your Diabetes...And Live a Healthy Life (Rogers Media Publishing, 2005).

Erhardt LR. 2005. Barriers to effective implementation of guideline recommendations. *Am J Med,* 118(12A):36S–41S.

Gluckman TJ et al. 2004. Taking LDL cholesterol to a new level. *Textbook of Cardiovascular Medicine Updates,* 7(2):1–16.

Gordon NF et al. 2004. Effectiveness of therapeutic lifestyle changes in patients with hypertension, hyperlipidemia, and/or hyperglycemia. *Am J Cardiol*, 94:1558–1561.

Guilliams TG. 2004. Homocysteine — A risk factor for vascular diseases: Guidelines for the clinical practice. *JAMA*, 7:11–24.

Gundry SM et al. 2004. Implications of recent clinical trials for the National Cholesterol Education Program Adult Treatment Panel III Guidelines. *J Am Coll Cardiol*, 44:720–732.

Hess P. 2005. Toward a new definition of hypertension. *The Cardiology Report*, 12:2 (Fall):5–11.

Hu FB et al. 2003. Television watching and other sedentary behaviors in relation to risk of obesity and type 2 diabetes mellitus in women. *JAMA*, 289:1785–1791.

Hu FB et al. 2001. Diet, lifestyle, and the risk of type 2 diabetes mellitus in women. *N Engl J Med*, 345:790–797.

Jain A. 2004. *What Works for Obesity*. London: BMJ Publishing Group, 4–62.

JAMA Author Instructions, 2001. Systeme International (SI) conversion factors for selected laboratory components. http://jama.ama-assn.org/content/vol295/issue1/images/data/103/DC6/JAMA_auinst_si.dtl

Johnson BD et al. 2006. Persistent chest pain predicts cardiovascular events in women without obstructive coronary artery disease: Results from the NIH-NHLBI sponsored Women's Ischemia Evaluation (WISE) study. *Eur Heart J*, 27:1408–1415.

Kapur NK et al. 2005. High density lipoprotein cholesterol: A new frontier in lipid management. *Textbook of Cardiovascular Medicine Updates*, 8(5):1–20.

Knowler WC et al. 2002. Reduction in the incidence of type 2 diabetes with lifestyle intervention or metformin. *N Engl J Med*, 346:393–403.

Kris-Etherton PM et al. 2002. Fish consumption, fish oil, omega-3 fatty acids, and cardiovascular disease. AHA Scientific Statement. *Circulation*, 106:2747–2757.

Kullo IJ & Ballantyne CM. 2005. Conditional risk factors for atherosclerosis. *Mayo Clin Proc*, 80:219–230.

Kung HC, Hoyert DL, Zu JQ, Murphy SL., Deaths: Final data for 2005. National vital statistics reports; vol 56 no 10. Hyattsville, MD: National Center for Health Statistics.

LaRosa JC et al. 2005. Treating to New Targets (TNT) Investigators: Intensive lipid lowering with atorvastatin in patients with stable coronary disease. *N Engl J Med,* 352:1425–1435.

Levy D et al. 1996. The progression from hypertension to congestive heart failure. *JAMA,* 275:1557–1562.

Lichtenstein AH et al. 2006. Diet and lifestyle recommendations revision 2006: A scientific statement from the American Heart Association Nutrition Committee. *Circulation,* 114:82–96.

Liu S et al. 2000. A prospective study of dietary glycemic load, carbohydrate intake, and risk of coronary heart disease in US women. *Am J Clin Nutr,* 71:1455–1461.

Ludwig DS & Ebbeling CB. 2001. Type 2 diabetes mellitus in children: Primary care and public health considerations. *JAMA,* 286:1427–1430.

Manson JE et al. 1999. A prospective study of walking as compared with vigorous exercise in the prevention of coronary heart disease in women. *N Engl J Med,* 341:650–658.

McKeown NM et al. 2002. Whole-grain intake is favorably associated with metabolic risk factors for type 2 diabetes and cardiovascular disease in the Framingham Offspring Study. *Am J Clin Nutr,* 76:390–398.

Meyer TE et al. 2006. Long-term caloric restriction ameliorates the decline in diastolic function in humans. *J Am Coll Cardiol,* 47:398–402.

Mosca L et al. 2004. Evidence-based guidelines for cardiovascular disease prevention in women. *Circulation,* 109:672–693.

Mosca L et al. 2004. Tracking women's awareness of heart disease: An American Heart Association national study. *Circulation,* 109:573–579.

Murray CJ et al. 2003. Effectiveness and costs of interventions to lower systolic blood pressure and cholesterol: A global and regional analysis on reduction of cardiovascular disease risk. *Lancet,* 361:717–725.

Mykkanen L et al. 1999. LDL size and risk of coronary heart disease in elderly men and women. *Arterioscler Thromb Vasc Biol,* 19:2742–2748.

Nissen SE. 2005. Halting the progression of atherosclerosis with intensive lipid lowering: Results from the Reversal of Atherosclerosis with Aggressive Lipid Lowering (REVERSAL) trial. *Am J Med,* 118(12A):22S–27S.

Nissen SE et al. 2005. Statin therapy, LDL cholesterol, C-reactive protein and coronary artery disease. *N Engl J Med,* 352(1):29–38.

O'Keefe JH et al. 2004. Optimal low-density lipoprotein is 50 to 70 mg/dL. Lower is better and physiologically normal. *J Am Coll Cardiol,* 43:2142–2146.

Pate RR et al. 1995. Physical activity and public health. A recommendation from the Centers for Disease Control and Prevention and the American College of Sports Medicine. *JAMA,* 273:402–407.

Pereira MA et al. 2004. Dietary fiber and risk of coronary heart disease: A pooled analysis of cohort studies. *Arch Intern Med,* 164:370–376.

Pereira MA et al. 2004. Effects of a low-glycemic load diet on resting energy expenditure and heart disease risk factors during weight loss. *JAMA,* 292:2482–2490.

Qayyum R & Schulman P. 2005. Iron and atherosclerosis. *Clin Cardiol,* 28:119–122.

Rexrode KM et al. 1998. Abdominal adiposity and coronary heart disease in women. *JAMA,* 280:1843–1848.

Ridker PM et al. 2005. A randomized trial of low-dose aspirin in the primary prevention of cardiovascular disease in women. *N Engl J Med,* 352:1293–1304.

Ridker PM et al. 2005. C-reactive protein levels and outcomes after statin therapy. *N Engl J Med,* 352(1):20–8.

Ridker PM et al. 2001. Measurement of C-reactive protein for the targeting of statin therapy in the primary prevention of acute coronary events. *N Engl J Med,* 344:1959–1965.

Ridker PM et al. 1998. C-reactive protein adds to the predictive value of total and HDL cholesterol in determining risk of first myocardial infarction. *Circulation,* 97:2007–2011.

Rimm EB et al. 1996. Vegetable, fruit, and cereal fiber intake and risk of coronary heart disease among men. *JAMA,* 275:447–451.

Roberts CK et al. 2006. Effect of a diet and exercise intervention on inflammatory/anti-inflammatory properties of HDL in men with cardiovascular risk factors. *J Appl Physiol*, January 10 [Epub ahead of print].

Schnyder G et al. 2001. Decreased rate of coronary restenosis after lowering of plasma homocysteine levels. *N Engl J Med*, 345:1563–1600.

Sharrett AR et al. 2001. Coronary heart disease prediction from lipoprotein cholesterol levels, triglycerides, lipoprotein (a), apolipoproteins A-I and B, and HDL density subfractions: The Atherosclerosis Risk in Communities (ARIC) study. *Circulation*, 104:1108–1113.

Shlipak MG et al. 2000. Estrogen and progestin, lipoprotein (a) and the risk of recurrent coronary heart disease events after menopause. *JAMA*, 283:1845–1852.

Tanasescu M et al. 2003. Physical activity in relation to cardiovascular disease and total mortality among men with type 2 diabetes. *Circulation*, 107:2392–2394.

Tanko LB et al. 2005. Enlarged waist combined with elevated triglycerides is a strong predictor of accelerated atherogenesis and related cardiovascular mortality in postmenopausal women. *Circulation*, 111:1883–1890.

Thompson GR & Gundry SM, eds. 2005. Role of plant stanol esters in cholesterol management: Enhancing the efficacy of diet and statin therapy. *Am J Cardiol*, 96(Suppl 1A):1D–54D.

Thompson PD et al. 2003. Exercise and physical activity in the prevention and treatment of atherosclerotic cardiovascular disease: A statement from the Council on Clinical Cardiology (Subcommittee on Exercise, Rehabilitation, and Prevention) and the Council on Nutrition, Physical Activity and Metabolism (Subcommittee on Physical Activity). *Circulation*, 107:3109–3116.

Toth PP. 2005. The "good cholesterol": High-density lipoprotein. *Circulation*, 111:e89–e91.

Tuomilehto J et al. 2001. Prevention of type 2 diabetes mellitus by changes in lifestyle among subjects with impaired glucose tolerance. *N Engl J Med*, 344:1343–1350.

Tzou WS et al. 2005. Increased subclinical atherosclerosis in young adults with metabolic syndrome. *J Am Coll Cardiol*, 46:457–463.

U.S. Department of Health and Human Services, Centers for Disease Control and Prevention. 1996. *Physical Activity and Health: A Report of the Surgeon General.* http://www.cdc.gov/nccdphp/srg/srg.htm

Van Horn L. 1997. Fiber, lipids, and coronary heart disease. A statement for healthcare professionals from the Nutrition Committee, American Heart Association. *Circulation,* 95:2701–2704.

Wackers FJT et al. 2004. Detection of silent myocardial ischemia in asymptomatic diabetic subjects. The DIAD study. *Diabetes Care,* 27:1954–1961.

Weber MA. 2005. Cardiovascular and metabolic consequences of obesity. *Textbook of Cardiovascular Medicine Updates,* 8:1–16.

Welch GN & Loscalzo J. 1998. Homocysteine and atherothrombosis. *N Engl J Med,* 338:1042–1050.

Wessel TR et al. 2004. Upgrading prevention in patients with coronary artery disease: emphasis on hypertension. *Textbook of Cardiovascular Medicine Updates,* 7(3):1–16.

White WB. 2005. Update on the drug treatment of hypertension in patients with cardiovascular disease. *Am J Med,* 118:695–705.

Wilson PWF et al. 2005. C-Reactive protein and risk of cardiovascular disease in men and women from the Framingham Heart Study. *Arch Intern Med,* 165:2473–2478.

Wing RR & Hill JO. 2001. Successful weight loss maintenance. *Annu Rev Nutr,* 21:323–341.

Yeh ETH. 2005. High-sensitivity C-reactive protein as a risk assessment tool for cardiovascular disease. *Clin Cardiol,* 28:408–412.

Yusuf S et al. 2005. Obesity and the risk of myocardial infarction in 27,000 participants from 52 countries, a case-control study. *Lancet,* 366:1640–1649.

Glossary

A

Aspirin (also known as acetylsalicylic acid or ASA) = A pain reliever (analgesic) and an anti-inflammatory (to reduce the body's reaction to minor injury). Aspirin also is an effective blood-thinning agent, which reduces risk of heart attacks.

Aerobic exercise = Exercise of moderate intensity undertaken for extended periods of time, the result of which strengthens muscles throughout the body, particularly those of the heart and those aiding respiration. Aerobic exercise can reduce a person's cardiovascular risk.

Alcohol consumption = Moderate drinking of alcohol (meaning one drink a day for women or smaller/elderly adults and two drinks a day for non-elderly men) may provide health benefits, including a reduction in cardiovascular risk. However, alcohol consumption is a classic "double-edged sword" because of the very narrow safety range; higher levels of daily drinking can lead to liver and heart disease as well as increased risks of accidents or injuries.

American College of Cardiology (ACC) = The professional medical society for cardiovascular specialists headquartered in Washington, DC.

American Heart Association (AHA) = A voluntary health organization dedicated primarily to cardiovascular research and public education headquartered in Dallas, Texas.

Aneurysm = A blood-filled widening (dilatation) or bulge concentrated in a single area that is caused by disease or a weakening of the blood vessel wall. Although treatable, this bulge can burst, causing excessive bleeding or death.

Angina (stable/unstable) = Chest pain or discomfort that is caused by an imbalance of blood supply and oxygen demand. Stable angina refers to pain that is felt during exertion that subsides when the activity ends, while unstable angina can occur suddenly without warning.

Angioplasty = A process to re-open or enlarge blood vessels that are closed or occluded. It may involve one of several techniques including expanding a small balloon in the vessel, injecting agents to dissolve clots, or inserting a metal device called a stent to keep the vessel open.

Antioxidant = Agents that inhibit oxidation, which can damage tissues, especially those involved in atherosclerosis, aging, and development of cancer. Various nutrients, vitamins, and minerals — such as vitamin C and beta carotene — contribute to antioxidant functions.

Artery = A thick-walled blood vessel that carries blood away from the heart. Almost all arteries contain red or oxygenated blood.

Atherosclerosis = The most common form of arteriosclerosis or "hardening of the arteries." Lipid deposits mix with various cells to become plaque, causing arteries to narrow; plaques can lead to calcification or "hardening," limiting or even stopping blood flow through the vessel.

B

Blood clot = A clump formed by blood coagulating and hardening from a liquid to a solid. A blood clot that forms in a blood vessel or the heart and remains there is called a thrombus; if the blood clot becomes free-floating and moves to another location in the body, it is called an embolus.

Blood pressure = The pressure exerted by the blood against the inner walls of the blood vessels, especially the arteries. It varies in different parts of the body during different phases of contraction of the heart as well as due to the strength of the heartbeat; other influences include the elasticity of the arterial walls; the volume of the blood; a person's health, age, and physical condition; and more. Blood pressure is expressed as two numbers: at its peak (systole) and at its lowest level during the resting phase of the cardiac cycle (diastole).

Blood sugar = The amount of glucose in the blood. Glucose serves as the primary source of energy for the body's cells. Poor regulation of glucose can lead to persistently high (hyperglycemia) or low (hypoglycemia) levels of blood sugar.

Blood vessels = A part of the cardiovascular system, blood vessels carry oxygen-rich blood away from the heart (in the arteries) and carry oxygen-depleted blood back to the heart (in the veins). The aorta is the largest artery in the body. While vessels do not actively transport blood, they can regulate their inner diameter by contracting their muscular layer; this can influence the amount of blood flow to organs.

Body mass index (BMI) = This number is calculated from a person's weight and height and provides a reliable indicator of body fatness. BMI can be used to screen for weight categories that may lead to health problems.

C

Carbohydrate = Carbohydrates are organic compounds that include sugars, starches, celluloses, and gums and serve as a major energy source in the diet. The simplest carbohydrates are the monosaccharides, which include the sugars glucose and fructose. The healthiest sources of carbohydrates are fruits, vegetables, and whole grains.

Cardiac cycle = The events related to the flow of blood that occur from the beginning of one heartbeat to the beginning of the next; heart rate measures the frequency of the cardiac cycle. The cycle is divided into two stages: diastole, when the heart's lower chambers, the ventricles, are filling followed by systole, the stage when these chambers contract ejecting blood.

Cardiomyopathy = Literally "heart muscle disease," this disease classification applies when function of the heart muscle (myocardium) deteriorates for any reason.

Cardiovascular disease = This refers to diseases involving the heart (cardio-) or blood vessels (-vascular). It is most often applied to conditions related to atherosclerosis; these have similar underlying causes, mechanisms, and treatments.

Cerebrovascular accident (CVA) = More commonly called a stroke, this is the sudden death of brain cells due to a lack of oxygen when blood flow is impaired due to blockage or a rupture of an artery to the brain.

Cholesterol = A fat-like, waxy substance, cholesterol is found in the cell membranes of all tissues and plays a role in many of the body's biochemical processes. It is transported in blood bound to one of a variety of lipoproteins. Abnormally high levels of cholesterol are associated with cardiovascular disease.

Cholesterol profile = Also called a lipid profile, this outlines the patterns of lipids in the blood, including measurements of total cholesterol, high-density lipoproteins (HDL), low-density lipoproteins (LDL), and triglycerides.

Cholesterol ratio = The ratio of total cholesterol to high-density lipoprotein (HDL) cholesterol. For example, if a person's total cholesterol is 200 mg/dL and HDL is 50 mg/dL, the cholesterol ratio is 4:1. Most physicians find the absolute numbers rather than the ratio provide more useful information to determine treatment for patients.

Chronic = Long-lasting; in medicine, the term may apply to the course of a disease or its rate of onset and development.

Computed tomography (CT) = A medical imaging technique that provides three-dimensional anatomic information from a series of two-dimensional X-ray images. Each image is generated by a computer synthesis of x-ray data obtained in many different directions (planes). Also called computed axial tomography or CAT scan.

Coronary artery bypass graft (CABG) surgery = Surgery in which a vein or artery from another part of the body is connected at points before and after a blockage in a coronary artery, "bypassing" the problem. Double, triple, quadruple, or quintuple bypass refers to the number of grafts to be implanted.

Coronary artery disease (CAD) = A spectrum of diseases of the heart, occurring when the arteries supplying the heart with oxygen and nutrients narrow and become blocked. CAD may lead to a heart attack, the need for CABG or angioplasty, or even sudden death. It is the most common cause of death in people over the age of 20 years.

C-reactive protein (cRP) = A protein found in blood plasma, levels of cRP rise in response to inflammation in the body.

D

Diabetes mellitus (type 1 and type 2) = A chronic metabolic disorder in which utilization of carbohydrates is impaired while utilization of lipids and proteins is enhanced. It is characterized by high blood sugar levels and inadequate insulin levels or sensitivity. Characteristic symptoms include excessive urine production, excessive thirst and increased fluid intake, and blurred vision. Type 1 is usually due to the destruction of insulin-producing cells in the pancreas, leading to reduced insulin levels, and patients must take insulin; thus, it is called insulin-dependent diabetes. Most people with type 1 diabetes develop it before age 30, which is why it is also called juvenile diabetes. In type 2 diabetes, the body becomes resistant to the effects of insulin; this form of diabetes can often be managed with dietary treatment and medication, although insulin supplementation may be needed. It also is known as adult-onset diabetes.

Diagnosis = Determining the nature of a disease, injury, or defect.

Diastole = The resting stage in the cardiac cycle or during a heartbeat when the ventricles, the heart's lower chambers, are filling with blood.

E

Edema = Swelling caused by fluids in the body. Heart failure is often accompanied by edema.

Endothelium = The cells that line the inner surface of all blood vessels.

Exercise = Physical activity to maintain fitness and health. Frequent and regular physical exercise boosts the immune system and helps prevent cardiovascular disease, type 2 diabetes, and obesity.

F

Family history = Information about a patient's direct relatives in terms of medical disorders and conditions the family members may have or have had to help determine a patient's risk of suffering the same disease (e.g., cardiovascular disease, diabetes, etc.).

Fasting blood glucose (FBG) = A measurement taken after fasting for at least eight hours; it measures how much sugar (glucose) is in the blood and is one of the first tests conducted to determine whether a patient has diabetes. Normal FBG is less than 100 mg/dL; a level of 100–125 mg/dL indicates the presence of prediabetes, and a level above 125 mg/dL usually indicates diabetes.

Fiber = The indigestible portions of plant food. Diets high in fiber have positive health benefits, including improved digestive health; improved glucose tolerance; reduction in coronary risk factors and high blood pressure; and lower risk of developing certain cancers. High-fiber diets also increase the sense of being full when eating and may help with weight management. The American Dietetic Association recommends a minimum of 20–35 grams of fiber per day for healthy adults.

Flavonoid = Compounds in fruits, vegetables, and some beverages such as wine that have beneficial antioxidant and biochemical effects. Research suggests that individuals whose diets are high in flavonoids reduce their risk of heart disease and cancer.

G

Gender = The sex of an individual (male or female).

Genetics = The field of science that studies heredity, or how traits are passed down from one generation to another through genes, which contain DNA and determine characteristics in organisms.

Glycosylated hemoglobin (HbA1c) = A form of hemoglobin used to identify a person's average plasma glucose (blood sugar) concentration over prolonged periods of time. It is used to check blood sugar control in individuals who are or might be prediabetic or diabetic.

H

Health and Human Services, U.S. Department of (HHS) = The U.S. government's principal agency for protecting health and providing human services. It includes more than 300 programs and departments that cover everything from health and social science research to Medicare and Head Start programs.

Heart failure (HF) = This condition results from any structural or functional cardiac disorders that impair the ability of the heart to fill with blood or pump blood sufficiently. As the blood flows more slowly out of the heart, blood returning to the heart (through veins) backs up, causing congestion. This is why the condition has been commonly called congestive heart failure (CHF). Heart failure is usually accompanied by swelling (edema). Heart failure also can impact the kidneys' ability to cleanse and eliminate sodium and water, increasing swelling. Because not all heart failure is congestive in nature, today it is often commonly referred to as chronic heart failure or just heart failure.

Hemoglobin = The protein in red blood cells that carries oxygen.

Heredity = The transfer of characteristics, including tendencies to develop certain conditions or diseases, from parent to children through their genes.

High-density lipoprotein (HDL) = Often called the "good" cholesterol, this complex of lipids and proteins are smaller in size but greater in density than LDL and carry fatty acids and cholesterol from body tissue to the liver for elimination. An HDL level of 60 mg/dL is considered protective of cardiovascular health; lower than 40 increases an increased risk of heart disease.

Homocysteine = An amino acid, homocysteine is a biomarker for cardiovascular disease — the higher the level of homocysteine the higher the risk of cardiovascular disease.

Hormone = A chemical substance carried in the blood from one organ or part of the body to another to regulate cell function. Different hormones have different effects, including regulating metabolism, activating or inhibiting the immune system, stimulating or inhibiting growth, inducing or suppressing cell death, and more.

Hypercholesterolemia = An excess of cholesterol in the blood that increases the risk of cardiovascular disease. Together with diet and exercise, physicians may prescribe lipid-lowering agents such as statins to lower the level of cholesterol.

Hyperglycemia = An abnormally high concentration of blood sugar (glucose), seen especially in diabetes.

Hyperlipidemia = An abnormally high presence of lipids and/or lipoproteins (cholesterol) in the blood.

Hypertension = High blood pressure defined as a systolic pressure above 140 mm/Hg or a diastolic pressure above 90 mm/Hg. Essential (or primary) hypertension indicates no known medical condition to explain the condition;

secondary hypertension means the high blood pressure is resulting from another condition such as kidney disease. Persistent hypertension is a risk factor for heart failure, heart attacks, strokes, and more. Lifestyle changes, including diet and physical activity, are often encouraged; a variety of medications can be prescribed to treat hypertension.

I

Incidence = The number of new occurrences of a specified condition or disease; for example, the number of women experiencing heart failure in 2007.

Inflammation = A nonspecific immune response, inflammation is the basic way the body reacts to infection, irritation, or injury. Risk factors that promote atherosclerosis such as cigarette smoking, hypertension, hyperglycemia, and plaque-causing fats (lipoproteins), all give rise to substances that release chemicals and activate cells involved in the inflammatory process.

Insulin = A hormone secreted by the pancreas, insulin is released when the body detects an increase in blood sugar. It binds to nearly every type of cell in the body to help cells absorb glucose for energy. Individuals with type 1 diabetes typically manufacture insulin poorly or not at all and must use supplemental insulin via shots or a pump.

Insulin resistance = Typical of type 2 diabetes, insulin resistance occurs when cells in the body do not respond normally to insulin and do not absorb enough glucose, which can elevate blood sugar levels.

Ischemia = Insufficient blood supply to a body part, usually due to blood vessel constriction or obstruction. Myocardial ischemia occurs when heart tissue is deprived of blood and the oxygen it carries. When blood flow is completely blocked to the heart, ischemia can lead to a heart attack (myocardial infarction).

L

Left ventricle = The main pumping chamber of the heart.

Life expectancy = A statistical measure of the average time of survival. The measure is highly dependent on the criteria used for the selected group. For example, life expectancy for populations in developing countries is usually far different than for those in industrialized nations.

Lifestyle factors = Aspects of daily living that can affect one's health and risk of cardiovascular and other diseases. These are often modifiable and include such things as diet, smoking and alcohol use, and level of physical activity.

Lipoprotein = Any compound containing both lipids and proteins. Many enzymes, transporters, antigens, and even toxins are lipoproteins. The more dense the lipoprotein, the more protein it contains versus fat. Thus high-density lipoproteins (HDL) have the most protein and least fat of these compounds.

Lipoprotein A (Lp(a)) = Composed of a low-density lipoprotein particle combined with an additional protein, Lp(a) is a risk factor for coronary artery disease.

Low-density lipoprotein (LDL) = Often called the "bad" cholesterol because high levels of LDL increases risk of atherosclerosis and cardiovascular disease. These lipoproteins are less dense than HDL and carry cholesterol from the liver to the cells of the body. Because the LDL can be retained in these cells, it can be the raw material from which plaques are formed. Optimally, LDL levels should be below 100 mg/dL; for patients with cardiovascular disease or those with diabetes, LDL should be 70 mg/dL or less.

Lumen = The space in any tubular structure. In a blood vessel, it is the open space through which blood flows.

M

Mediterranean diet = A diet that reduces the risk of cardiovascular disease built around the eating habits of most cultures living near the Mediterranean Sea. It includes high consumption of fruits, vegetables, breads, cereals, potatoes, and beans; the use of healthy fats such as olive and canola oils; eating small amounts of nuts; very little consumption of red meat; eating more moderate amounts of dairy, poultry, fish, and eggs; and drinking wine (preferably red) in small to moderate amounts.

Metabolic syndrome = A combination of risk factors that increase a person's risk of cardiovascular disease or diabetes. These factors include abdominal obesity (excessive fat tissue in and around the abdomen), insulin resistance or glucose intolerance, high blood pressure, low HDL, and higher triglycerides. Individuals with metabolic syndrome have higher circulating levels of prothrombotic and proinflammatory markers, increasing their risk of cardiovascular disease.

Metabolism = The entire range of biochemical processes within living organisms necessary to maintain life. This includes both the production and breakdown or transformation of substances into energy or products used by the body. Commonly used to refer to the breakdown of food and its transformation into energy.

Myocardial infarction (MI) = Commonly known as a "heart attack," an MI occurs when blood flow to the heart is interrupted; the resulting shortage of oxygen causes damage or even death of heart tissue. The term comes from myocardium (heart muscle) and infarction (tissue death due to oxygen starvation). Symptoms include chest tightness or pain (that may radiate to the left arm), shortness of breath, nausea, vomiting, sweating, palpitations, and anxiety; women may experience different symptoms from men.

N

National Institutes of Heath (NIH) = A part of the U.S. Department of Health and Human Services, NIH is the primary federal agency for conducting and supporting medical research. It is composed of 27 institutes and centers; NIH research conducted on cardiovascular and related diseases is under the auspices of the National Heart, Lung, and Blood Institute.

O

Obese = Weighing more than 20 percent above the weight considered normal for height, age, gender, and build. National Institutes of Health defines obesity as a body mass index of 30 and above; a BMI of 30 equals about 30 pounds overweight.

Omega-3 fatty acid = A family of polyunsaturated acids that may help reduce a person's risk of cardiovascular disease. Available as a dietary supplement, omega-3 fatty acids also are found in fish, flax, various berries and fruits, some nuts, and eggs.

Overweight = Weighing more than is healthy or normal for one's age, height, and build. Defined as a body mass index of 25 to 30.

Oxygen = The essential element in the respiration process of living beings. Oxygen is carried in the hemoglobin of red blood cells.

P

Pathophysiology = Study of the changes associated with or resulting from disease or injury; also considered the study of the manifestations of disease.

Peripheral vascular disease (PVD) = Diseases of the blood vessels outside the heart and brain. Many PVDs are due to structural changes in the blood vessel. The most common PVD is peripheral arterial disease (PAD), which is similar to coronary artery disease because fatty deposits/plaques build up along the arterial wall. Other PVDs are not due to any structural change in the vessel. For example, Raynaud's disease is a PVD in which blood vessels excessively narrow due to cold temperatures.

Plaque = Sticky deposits that build up in the inner lining of an artery. The presence of plaque is called atherosclerosis and it can lead to heart disease and stroke.

Platelet = A type of blood cell (also called a thrombocyte) that prevents bleeding by causing the formation of blood clots after an injury. Low levels of platelets may lead to increased bleeding; high levels of platelets may cause harmful clots to form in the blood.

Postmenopausal = The period of life after a woman has ceased having menstrual periods for 12 consecutive months. The change in hormone levels puts women at risk for various diseases. Once commonly treated with hormone replacement therapy, this approach is more controversial today given evidence that such therapy can increase risk of developing heart disease.

Prediabetes = A state in which blood glucose levels are higher than normal but not yet high enough to be considered diabetes. It is thought to be a precursor to type 2 diabetes.

Prehypertension = A newly recognized state in which blood pressure levels are between 120 mm/Hg systolic and 80 mm/Hg diastolic (normal blood pressure) and 139/89 mm Hg, which is not yet high enough to be labeled hypertension but is likely to progress to hypertension without treatment or intervention.

Prevalence = The measure of a condition or the number of cases of a disease in a population at a given point in time.

Progression = The advancement or growth of a disease, with or without treatment.

Pulse pressure = The difference between the highest (systole) and lowest (diastole) blood pressure readings, pulse pressure represents the force that the heart generates each time it contracts. A person with a blood pressure reading 125/83 mm Hg would have a pulse pressure of 42 mm/Hg.

R

Regression = When symptoms or a disease subside; a return to an earlier state.

Revascularization = The act of restoring blood flow to a part of the body. Coronary revascularization restores blood flow with procedures such as angioplasty or coronary artery bypass graft surgery.

Risk factor = Any variable that increases a person's chance of developing a disease. Some risk factors may be modifiable (weight, level of physical activity); others may be treatable (high blood pressure, diabetes); while still others are not modifiable (age, gender).

S

Saturated fat = Solid at room temperature, these fats do not combine readily with oxygen and are a main dietary factor in raising cholesterol levels. The primary source of saturated fat in the typical American diet is from animal fats.

Serologic markers = Markers that are found in serum, the clear yellowish fluid obtained upon separating whole blood into its solid and liquid components. These markers are used to distinguish specific diseases in individuals, especially useful in the early stages of disease before symptoms are present. Also, may be used to confirm the diagnosis of an acute heart attack.

Sleep apnea = Pauses in breathing (apnea) of at least 10 seconds between breaths while one is sleeping. The lack of quality sleep (sleep deprivation) and lack of oxygen caused by sleep apnea can increase risk of developing cardiovascular disease, high blood pressure, stroke, diabetes, and weight gain.

Sodium = The primary electrolyte that helps maintain water balance in the body and assists with other functions. However, too much sodium in the diet can lead to high blood pressure. Healthy adults should have less than 2,400 mg of sodium a day; that is the amount in one teaspoon of table salt.

Stenosis = A constricting or narrowing of a blood vessel.

Strength training = Exercise program that strengthens muscles that uses the force of gravity against the force generated by the muscle. This type of exercise can help improve cardiovascular health.

Stress test = A medical test that evaluates blood flow to the heart. The heart is stressed by performing exercise, such as running on a treadmill, or by administration of a medication that speeds (or "stresses") the heart in a simulation of exercise, while various measurements are taken, such as blood pressure or an electrocardiogram.

Stroke = Rapid loss of brain function due to a disturbance in the blood vessels supplying blood to the brain. A stroke may be caused by an embolism, a clot that has traveled to the brain and blocks a blood vessel, or a hemorrhage, which is excessive bleeding in the space between the brain and the skull.

Systole = The stage in the cardiac cycle or during a heart beat when the ventricles, the heart's lower chambers, contract and eject the blood in them.

T

Thrombosis = Clotting within a blood vessel that can cause the death of tissue due the lack of oxygen-rich blood.

Total cholesterol = A measurement of all cholesterols in the blood. A level less than 200 mg/dL is desirable, 200–239 mg/dL is considered borderline high risk, and 240 mg/dL and above is considered high risk.

Trans fats = Common name for chemically modified ("hydrogenated" or "partially hydrogenated") unsaturated fats. Trans fats raise LDL cholesterol levels and lower HDL cholesterol levels. These are neither required in the diet nor beneficial for health, and eating trans fats can increase the risk of cardiovascular disease.

Triglyceride = Chemical form in which most fats exist in the body. Triglycerides are present in blood plasma and form plasma lipids with cholesterol. High triglyceride levels increase the risk of coronary artery disease, although the association is not as powerful as for LDL elevation.

U

Unsaturated fat = Usually liquid at room temperature, unsaturated fats generally come from vegetarian sources. Monounsaturated and polyunsaturated fats are both included in this group. Unsaturated fat is a healthier alternative to saturated fat and can be found in vegetable oils such as canola, sesame, sunflower, and olive; oily fish, such as sardines, herring and salmon; as well as nuts and avocados.

V

Vasoconstriction = Narrowing of the lumen or inner space of blood vessels, which can restrict blood flow; vasoconstriction can result from medications or substances such as caffeine or disease.

Vasodilation = Widening of the lumen of the blood vessel due to relaxation of the muscular wall of the vessel.

Very low-density lipoprotein cholesterol (VLDL-C) = These lipoproteins transport triglycerides from the intestines and liver to muscles and tissues.

W

White-coat hypertension = Elevated blood pressure that occurs only in the doctor's office; appears related to nervousness about the appointment as opposed to an underlying condition or problem that causes chronic blood pressure elevation.

Index

A

ACC. *See* American College of Cardiology

Acetylsalicylic acid. *See* Aspirin

Adrenaline
  stress and, 170
  symptoms of rises in, 173-174

Adult-onset diabetes. *See* Pre-diabetes; Type 2 diabetes

Aerobic exercise
  description, 207

Age factors
  cholesterol level, 32
  hypertension, 82
  insulin balance and, 101
  low-density lipoprotein, 50
  pulse pressure, 77
  stress, 170
  type 2 diabetes, 103

AHA. *See* American Heart Association

Alcohol consumption
  effect of using mixes and additives, 42
  high-density lipoprotein level and, 40, 41-42
  hypertension and, 28, 81-82
  low-density lipoprotein and, 49
  moderate, 28, 40, 41-42, 81-82, 207
  "one drink" description, 42
  stress and, 174
  wine, 42

American College of Cardiology. *See also* CardioSmart
  description and activities, v-vi, 207
  goals of the book, xii-xiv, 3
  legal issues concerning the book, xiii-xiv

American Heart Association
  description and activities, 207

American Lung Association
  resource for quitting smoking, 95

Aneurysms
  description, 207
Angina
  description, 208
  stress and, 174
  symptoms, 182
Angioplasty
  description, 208
Animal protein. *See* Saturated fats
Antioxidant
  description, 208
Artery
  description, 208
ASA. *See* Aspirin
Aspirin
  C-reactive protein and, 72
  complications from, 21
  daily therapy, 21
  description and mechanism of action, 21, 207
  preventive dose, 21
Atherosclerosis
  C-reactive protein and, 65, 71-72, 73
  description, 10, 208
  elevated blood sugar levels and, 101
  homocysteine level and, 70, 73, 188
  lipoprotein A testing and, 69
  low-density lipoprotein and, 48
  stroke and, 22
  systemic nature of, 22

B

Bad cholesterol. *See* Low-density lipoprotein
Baked goods
  recommendations for eating, 130-131
Beans and legumes
  recommendations for eating, 137, 191

Beef
saturated fats and, 138
Berries
benefits of eating, 134
Beverages. *See* Fluids
Blood clots
description, 208
endothelium injury and, 17-19
lipoprotein A and, 64
progress of, 18
women and, 180
Blood pressure. *See also* Hypertension
description, 208-209
normal values, 76, 79, 189
Blood pressure diaries, 87, 89
Blood sugar. *See also* Diabetes; Pre-diabetes
description, 209
frequency of evaluations for, 106
glycosylated hemoglobin test, 106-108
health effects of elevated levels, 100, 101-102
high-fiber diet and, 132
importance of knowing, 105
normal fasting blood glucose, 100, 103, 199
oral glucose tolerance test, 103-104
stress effects on, 170
symptoms of elevated blood sugar, 106
Blood tests. *See* Serologic markers; *specific tests*
Blood vessels. *See also* Coronary arteries
description, 209
BMI. *See* Body Mass Index
Body Mass Index
description, 114, 209
formula for, 114
normal values, 116, 190-191
obesity and overweight and, 113, 290
tables, 115
Bread. *See also* Baked goods

long-term weight control and, 151
low-density lipoprotein and, 49, 50, 73
lunch, 124
normal eating, 117-118
portion control, 120-121, 191
quality versus quantity, 114, 122-123, 149
snacking, 123-124, 126, 191
stress and, 174
summary of recommendations, 150
triglycerides and, 55, 56, 73
type 2 diabetes and, 98, 104
visualization exercise, 151
Dinner
late-night snacking and, 123-124
portions for, 123-124
Dried fruits
recommendations for eating, 134
Drinking. *See* Alcohol consumption

E

Eating habits. *See* Diet
Eating out. *See* Restaurants
Edema
description, 212
Eggs
benefits of eating, 143
cholesterol and, 142-143
Endothelium
blood clots and, 17-19
description, 16, 212
neck and brain arteries and, 22
plaque buildup and vulnerability of, 16-17, 65
risk factors for vulnerability of, 20, 21
smoking and, 92
stress and, 171
stroke and, 22, 65

Flavonoids
  description, 212-213
Flaxseed oil
  nonsaturated fat source, 140
Fluids
  fruit and vegetable juices, 133, 135, 148
  hot beverages, 148-149
  water, 148, 191
Folate. *See* Folic acid
Folic acid
  homocysteine level and, 64-65, 70-71
Fruits
  berries, 134
  canned types, 144
  creating dishes with, 134-135
  dried fruits, 134
  general recommendations, 133, 191
  number of daily servings, 134
  organic types, 133
  serving size, 133, 134
  snacking on, 126
  whole fruits versus fruit juice, 133

G

Gender. *See also* Men; Women's issues
  description, 213
Genetic factors
  cholesterol level, 33, 166
  diabetes, 164
  family health history and, 165-167, 192
  heart disease, 164, 192
  importance of knowing your genetic makeup, 163-164
  low-density lipoprotein, 49
  prevention issues, 166-167
  stroke, 164
  triglycerides, 56

type 2 diabetes, 103

Genetics
  description, 213

Glucose level. *See* Blood sugar

Glycosylated hemoglobin test
  description, 106-107, 213
  importance of, 107
  normal levels, 107

Good cholesterol. *See* High-density lipoprotein

Green tea
  benefits of, 148, 149

Gunk. *See* Plaque

H

HbA1c. *See* Glycosylated hemoglobin test

HDL. *See* High-density lipoprotein

Heart attacks
  atypical symptoms of heart attacks in women, 182, 193
  blood clots and, 17-19
  bypass surgery and stent treatments, 186
  C-reactive protein and, 65
  compared with stroke, 22
  description, 217
  heart muscle death and, 23-24
  low-density lipoprotein and, 45, 46, 47
  mild and moderate artery blockages and, 13, 16
  normal stress tests and, 20, 186
  pre-hypertension and, 77
  severe artery blockages and, 13
  stress and, 171, 192
  symptoms, 182
  systole effects, 27
  women and, 180, 181, 182

Heart disease. *See also* Coronary artery disease
  diabetes and, 101-102, 181-182

additional blood work and, 70

daily multivitamin supplements and, 65

description, 64, 188, 214

folic acid, vitamin B6, and vitamin B12 and, 64-65, 70-71

heart disease and, 71, 188

normal levels of, 64, 199

personal or family history of atherosclerosis and, 70, 73, 188

Hormonal supplementation

benefits and risks, 38, 193

heart disease and, 181, 193

using the lowest effective dose, 181

Hormones

description, 214

Hypercholesterolemia

description, 214

Hyperglycemia

description, 214

Hyperlipidemia

description, 214

Hypertension. *See also* Pulse pressure

alcohol consumption and, 28

blood pressure diaries, 87, 89

C-reactive protein and, 72

causes, 80-81

description, 27, 214-215

diabetes and, 28

diastolic value, 76, 189

estimated number of people affected by, 75-76

exercise and, 27-28, 70, 81, 83

goals for normal blood pressure, 76-78

heart disease and, 78, 79, 189

heart failure and, 27, 78, 80, 189

home blood pressure monitors and, 79, 86-87, 88, 189

lifestyle issues, 29, 80-81, 86, 189

medications to lower, 79, 88, 189

metabolic syndrome and, 55, 187

description, 215

Intermediate-density lipoprotein. *See* Non-HDL cholesterol

Ischemia
 description, 215

J

Juices
 fruit juice, 133, 148, 191
 serving size, 133, 148
 vegetable juice, 135, 148

Juvenile diabetes. *See* Type 1 diabetes

K

Kidney disease
 pulse pressure and, 77

Kidneys
 stress and, 171

L

LDL. *See* Low-density lipoprotein

Left ventricle
 description, 216

Legumes. *See* Beans and legumes

Life expectancy
 description, 216
 diabetes and, 103
 heart disease and, 6
 obesity and, 110
 smoking and, 95
 stress and, 176

Lifestyle issues
 C-reactive protein and, 72
 cholesterol level and, 33, 187
 cumulative effects of, 2-3
 description, 216
 hypertension and, 29, 80-81, 86, 189

imparting healthful habits to children, 14
list of good lifestyle choices, 3-4, 194
living your life as if you already have heart disease, 13
low-density lipoprotein and, 49, 50, 187
motivation to make changes, 12, 24
pre-hypertension and, 77
struggling with, 195
triglycerides and, 55, 57, 58, 187
type 2 diabetes, 102
Lipoprotein
  description, 216
Lipoprotein A
  description, 63-64, 188, 216
  family or personal history of atherosclerosis and, 69
  monitoring levels of, 70, 73
  niacin therapy, 69-70
  normal levels of, 64, 199
Liver
  cholesterol and, 31, 33
  stress and, 171
Low-density lipoprotein
  artery blockages and, 45
  C-reactive protein and, 72
  calculating, 35
  cholesterol ratio, 50-51, 187
  current published recommendations, 48, 198
  description, 34, 45, 58, 187, 216
  fish oil supplements and, 142
  genetic issues, 49
  HDL-LDL relationship, 50-51
  heart attacks and, 45, 46, 47
  heart disease risk factors and, 48
  high-fiber diet and, 132
  ideal levels, 46, 58, 187, 198
  insulin and, 34, 45
  lipoprotein A level and, 70
  medications for lowering, 46, 49-50

methods for lowering, 49-50

milligram/deciliter (mg/dL) specification description, 62

more aggressive goals, 48

nonsaturated fats and, 139

particle size importance, 62-63

plaque buildup and, 46-47

saturated fats and, 138

stress and, 170

stroke and, 45, 46, 47, 48

sub fraction analysis, 63, 69, 73, 188

toxicity of, 45, 64

trans fats and, 141

triglycerides and, 54-55

Low-saturated-fat diet

triglycerides and, 56

Lp(a). *See* Lipoprotein A

Lumen

description, 216

Lunch

portions for, 124

M

Mediterranean diet

description, 217

Men. *See also* Women's issues

alcohol consumption and, 42

compared with women on health issues, 180, 193

high HDL level and, 38

Menopause

cholesterol level and, 33

hormonal supplementation and, 38, 180-181

low-density lipoprotein and, 50

Metabolic syndrome

description, 55, 58, 187, 217

fish oil supplements and, 142

heart disease and, 58

Metabolism
  description, 217
MI. *See* Heart attacks
Moderate alcohol consumption
  description, 28, 42, 207
  high-density lipoprotein level and, 40, 41-42
  hypertension and, 28, 81-82
Mortality
  heart disease, x, 5-6, 7, 24, 185
  obesity, 110
  smoking, 91, 92
Myocardial infarction. *See* Heart attacks

N

National Institutes of Health
  description, 218
Niacin
  lipoprotein A levels and, 69-70
NIH. *See* National Institutes of Health
Non-HDL cholesterol
  description, 66, 223
  formula for calculating, 67
  hidden nature of, 66
  ideal levels of, 67
  identifying patients at risk for heart disease and, 67
Nonsaturated fats. *See also* Saturated fats
  cholesterol and, 139
  description, 139, 222
  dietary sources, 139
  flax oil, 140
Nutrition. *See* Diet
Nuts
  health benefits, 140
  serving size, 140

O

Obesity. *See also* Overweight; Weight issues
  Body Mass Index and, 113, 114-116, 190
  calories in versus calories out and, 113
  description, 218
  exercise and, 114
  factors in, 111-112
  food cost and, 112-113
  food quality versus food quantity and, 114
  health effects, 113
  hypertension and, 27, 28, 79, 189
  life expectancy and, 110
  maps showing increase in, 111
  metabolic syndrome and, 55, 187
  mortality from, 110
  portion size and, 114, 191
  waist measurement and, 113, 116, 191
Omega-3 fatty acids
  amount to include in your diet, 141
  benefits of, 140
  description, 218
  dietary sources, 141
  fish oil supplements, 141-142
Oral glucose tolerance test
  description, 103-104
Osteocalcin
  exercise and, 154
Overweight
  biochemical imbalance and, 99, 100, 101
  Body Mass Index and, 113, 114-116, 290
  calories in versus calories out and, 113, 118
  description, 218
  diabetes and, 181
  diet effect on long-term weight control, 151
  eating less and moving more and, 113, 118
  exercise and, 114, 154, 156

R

Reduced-carbohydrate foods
  sweeteners and, 131
Refined or processed foods
  carbohydrates and, 127
  fiber and, 132
  sodium and, 84, 144
  trans fats and, 141
Regression
  description, 220
Restaurants
  avoiding extra bread at meals, 123
  business meals, 122, 124
  consumers' effect on the nutritional value of meals, 152
  fast-food restaurants, 141, 144, 147
  portion size and, 120, 121
Revascularization
  description, 220
Rice
  balancing with vegetables and lean protein, 129
  brown rice compared with white rice, 127, 128
Risk factors. *See also specific factors and disorders*
  cumulative effects of, 2-3
  description, 220
  endothelium vulnerability and, 17, 18, 20, 21
  heart attack prevention and, 20
  list of, 15, 20, 186
  stress effect on risk-factor control, 170

S

Salt. *See* Sodium consumption
Saturated fats. *See also* Nonsaturated fats
  description, 138, 220
  fish and, 139
  meats and, 138

recommended number of servings of animal protein per day, 139

Serologic markers. *See also specific tests*
 asking your doctor about, 68
 for cholesterol components, 61-74
 description, 220
 heart disease, 188

Sleep apnea
 description, 221
 heart failure and, 82-83
 hypertension and, 79, 82-83, 189
 symptoms, 82, 83

Small vessel disease
 women and, 180

SmokEnders
 resource for quitting smoking, 95

Smoking
 cancer and, 93
 "cold turkey" quitting, 93
 gradual process of quitting, 93-94
 heart disease and, 91, 95
 high-density lipoprotein level and, 40, 41
 hypertension and, 79, 81, 189
 importance of quitting, 91, 190
 life expectancy and, 95
 low-density lipoprotein and, 49
 mortality from, 91
 physical effects of tobacco smoke, 92
 resources for quitting, 95, 96
 resuming after quitting, 96
 secondhand smoke effects, 92
 stress and, 174
 vasoconstriction and, 81

Snacking
 compared with grazing, 126
 dangers of, 126
 foods to snack on, 126

professional help for, 176, 177, 192
risk-factor control and, 170
sources of, 173
strategies for dealing with, 175-177
support networks and, 173, 176
understanding your sources and levels of, 175
Stress tests
coronary artery blockage and, 12, 18, 20
description, 221
heart attacks and, 20, 186
Stroke
C-reactive protein and, 65
compared with heart attacks, 22
description, 22, 210, 221
fish oils and, 139
genetic factors, 164
hypertension and, 78
low-density lipoprotein and, 45, 46, 48
stress and, 171
Sub fraction analysis
high-density lipoprotein, 63, 69, 73, 188
low-density lipoprotein, 63, 69, 73, 188
Systole
description, 26, 221
heart damage due to heart attack and, 27
hypertension and, 27

T

Tea
benefits of drinking, 148-149, 191
green tea, 148
herbal teas, 148-149
Terminology, xiii, 207-223
TGs. *See* Triglycerides
Thrombosis
description, 222

risk factors, 103
routine testing and, 98

U

Unsaturated fats. *See* Nonsaturated fats
U.S. Department of Health and Human Services
  description, 213
  "My Family History Portrait," 165

V

Vasoconstriction
  description, 222
  smoking and, 81
Vasodilation
  description, 223
Vegetables
  building a meal around, 136
  canned types, 144
  eating a variety of, 135-136, 191
  as the foundation of your diet, 135
  general recommendations, 133, 191
  number of daily servings, 135
  portion size, 136
  potatoes, 135, 136
  salads, 136
  serving size, 135
  snacking on, 126
  soups, 137
  vegetable juices, 135
Very-low-density lipoprotein. *See* Non-HDL cholesterol
Vitamin B6
  homocysteine level and, 64-65, 70-71
Vitamin B12
  homocysteine level and, 64-65, 70-71
VLDL. *See* Non-HDL cholesterol

W

Waist circumference
  obesity and overweight and, 113, 116, 191
Walking
  calorie expenditure and, 158
  the fifteen-minute mile, 157-158
  incorporating into your daily activities, 157
  number of steps needed daily, 160
  treadmills and, 158
Water
  benefits of drinking, 148, 191
Weight issues. *See also* Obesity; Overweight
  C-reactive protein and, 72
  cholesterol level and, 33-34, 73
  high-density lipoprotein level, 40, 41
  hypertension, 27, 81, 189
  low-density lipoprotein, 49
  triglycerides, 55, 56-57
  type 2 diabetes, 98, 104
"White coat" hypertension
  description, 87, 223
Wine
  benefits from drinking, 42
Women's issues. *See also* Men
  alcohol consumption, 42
  atypical symptoms of heart attacks, 182, 193
  cholesterol level, 33
  compared with men on health issues, 180, 193
  diabetes, 181-182, 193
  HDL levels, 37, 38
  heart attacks, 180, 182
  heart disease, 6, 180, 181-183, 193
  hormonal supplementation and, 33, 38, 180-181, 193
  menopause, 33, 38, 180-181
  risk factors and, 179, 193
  small vessel disease, 180
  type 2 diabetes, 103